Child Care Law for Health Professionals

Judith Hendrick
Senior Lecturer in Law
Oxford Brookes University

With a Foreword by
Richard Williams
Consultant Child and Adolescent Psychiatrist
Bristol Royal Hospital for Sick Children

RADCLIFFE MEDICAL PRESS●OXFORD and NEW YORK

To Josie and Eve with love and for SB

©1993 Radcliffe Medical Press Ltd
15 Kings Meadow, Ferry Hinksey Road, Oxford OX2 0DP

Radcliffe Medical Press Inc, 141 Fifth Avenue, Suite N, New York, NY 10010, USA

British Library Cataloguing in Publication Data

A cataloguing record for this book is available from the British Library.

ISBN 1 870905 29 6

Typeset by Advance Typesetting Ltd, Oxfordshire
Printed and bound in Great Britain

Contents

Foreword

The Children Act 1989 has brought about the most significant change in the law relating to children and adolescents in England and Wales this century. This reflects not only mounting concern about the experience and treatment of certain children in the last quarter of the twentieth century but, also, fundamental changes in the position and status of children in our society over a much longer time-scale.

The Children Act has brought together much of the previous private and public law and updated it to encompass the spirit of a number of judgements made by the Courts. This Act offers a legal structure which recognizes and builds on the paramountcy of the welfare of children and, more clearly than ever before, identifies their rights whilst supporting the central position and responsibilities of families in their upbringing. A clear conception of partnership between families and services, particularly for those in adversity, is contained within this structure as is the improved integration of services. It is most appropriate, then, that this book should consider in detail the provisions of the Children Act and all the Regulations and Guidance published in relation to it.

The importance of this book is that it particularly considers child care law as it affects the role and practice of health care professionals. In the past, little training has been offered to the health service staff in this respect and my own under- and postgraduate experiences have exemplified this omission. I had to struggle, largely unaided, to familiarize myself with those aspects of the law which affected my practice. This text seizes on the opportunity presented by the enaction of the Children Act to fill this gap and it is a privilege for me to write this Foreword.

Written by a lawyer, this book covers interpretation of the law in detail but is clearly and concisely written, sensitive to demanding health care issues and the core points are richly illustrated by case examples. Readers will learn an enormous amount. I am certain that they will gain understanding, and greater comfort with potentially complex issues, which will contribute to the improved care of children through the more effective enaction in practice of the principles which lie behind recent legislation.

Richard Williams
Consultant Child and Adolescent Psychiatrist
Bristol Royal Hospital for Sick Children
September 1993

1

Introduction

Origins of the Act

When the Children Act came into force in October 1991, it was hailed as the most comprehensive reform in living memory and one which would bring about a new beginning to the philosophy and practices of the child care system. It was the outcome of a lengthy process of extensive consultation and debate and was influenced by a number of different factors.

The reform process began in the early 1980s with a comprehensive examination of children in care by a House of Commons Social Services Select Committee. This led to the publication in 1985 of the DHSS *Review of Child Care Law* – an ambitious document containing over 200 recommendations, most of which (but by no means all) were accepted by the Government and formed the basis of their 1987 White Paper: The Law on Child Care and Family Services.

At about the same time an equally comprehensive review of the private law of children was being carried out by the Law Commission. Its findings were published in a series of reports between 1984–8 and, perhaps not surprisingly given that the existing framework was found to be 'too complicated, confusing and largely unintelligible', radical reforms were recommended. Although these major reviews were crucial in providing a unique opportunity to harmonize reforms of virtually all child law, other reports also formed part of the background to the legislation. Notable amongst these were a series of highly publicized child abuse public inquiries.

Between 1980 and 1989 there were 18 reports into the death of children known to (and often in the care of) Social Services Departments. In most of these reports social workers were criticized for failing to use their statutory powers in time to 'save' children at risk. However, it was undoubtedly the 1987 Cleveland crisis which generated the most interest, forcing the problem of child sexual abuse into public debate and exposing the vulnerability of inter-agency systems. A particularly explosive element in the crisis was a major difference of medical opinion about the techniques for determining whether sexual abuse had occurred. Equally contentious was the role of social workers who were accused of acting precipitately and insensitively in removing nearly 100 children unnecessarily from their homes.

Another important influence on the legislation – but more difficult to assess – was the impact of such pressure groups as Family Rights Group, Parents Against Injustice, Justice for Children and the Children's Legal Centre. Similarly professional organizations like the British Association of Social Workers and the British Agencies for Adoption and Fostering were significant in the influence they exerted both in individual cases and on the policy-making process.

Finally, there was the landmark 1986 Gillick case from which is derived the phrase 'Gillick competent'. This upheld the right of girls under 16 to consent to contraceptive treatment without their parents' knowledge or consent. In doing so it recognized the rights of older children to autonomy and self-determination provided they had sufficient maturity and understanding to make up their own minds on a particular issue. It also acknowledged that a child's decision could supercede parental rights in matters of upbringing.

Scope of the Act

The Act is divided into 12 separate parts and has 108 sections and 15 schedules, and applies to England and Wales (with the exception of Part X, which also applies to Scotland). The schedules contain important supplemental matters of detail and have exactly the same legal effect as the sections. The Act includes both 'private' and 'public' law – terms which are not actually used in the legislation but which are commonly used by practitioners. Private law covers private disputes about children, for example, their living arrangements following divorce, child abduction, paternity issues and child maintenance. Public law deals with intervention in children's lives by public authorities. It therefore includes compulsory intervention by social services departments, as well as the voluntary provision of services and the regulation of substitute care, ie fostering and child-minding.

The following is a brief summary of the Act:

Part I: General principles

Part I affects both private and public law. It sets out the Act's fundamental principles and the provisions the courts must apply when deciding cases. These are the welfare and non-intervention principle, the welfare 'check list', the presumption against delay and the new concept of 'parental responsibility'. Guardianship law is also amended and simplified.

Part II: Orders in family proceedings

Part II introduces a new range of court orders – collectively called Section 8 orders – which are most likely to be used to resolve disputes between private individuals when they cannot agree about various aspects of a child's upbringing. Nevertheless, these orders can in some circumstances be used by local authorities and health authorities. The new scheme also considerably improves the legal standing of children, unmarried fathers and other relatives, giving them greater rights to initiate court proceedings.

Part III: Local authority services

This Part is concerned with public law. It contains the main provisions covering local authorities' duties to safeguard and promote the welfare of children (primarily those defined as 'in need'), by preventing family breakdown and providing a range of support and preventive services. Although these services remain very similar to those available under previous law, the statutory framework has been recast so as to present service provision in a more positive, less stigmatizing way. It incorporates a 'partnership' model of practice between parents, children, local authorities and other agencies. Part III also specifies the duties owed by local authorities to children they are looking after.

Parts IV and V: Care, supervision and child protection

Both these Parts are concerned with compulsory state intervention. Part IV sets out the new criteria for care proceedings (no longer available for 'truanting' children or those facing criminal proceedings) and supervision proceedings. The court's powers to regulate contact with children in care are also substantially reformed as are the duration and effect of both full and interim orders. Part V introduces new provisions for the protection of children at risk of harm either in emergency situations or less urgent cases where a medical assessment of the child is the priority. The investigative responsibilities of local authorities are likewise amended. Finally, Part V includes police powers and other provisions concerning abducted and missing children.

Parts VI, VII and VIII: Children's homes

Parts VI, VII and VIII contain provisions concerning the welfare of children who are looked after outside the family home. They cover the provision, management and conduct of various types of children's homes, whether provided by the local authority or private sector, and aim to ensure that uniform standards apply to all facilities.

Part IX: Private fostering

This Part regulates 'private' fostering arrangements (those not arranged by local authorities). Whilst much of the old law is simply repeated, some terminological changes have been introduced and the supervisory powers and duties of local authorities have been clarified.

Part X: Child-minding and day care

The registration and regulation of child-minding and day care services for children under the age of eight years old are covered here. Existing law is modified and updated to reflect recent developments in childcare provision. Overall the reforms aim to facilitate local authority control over services.

Part XI: The role of the Secretary of State

This Part lists the supervisory functions of the Secretary of State and includes the inspection of premises, research funding and training.

Part XII: Miscellaneous

Part XII includes new provisions on paternity testing, legal aid, appeals and adoption law and creates a new framework to protect children living in health and educational establishments, private nursing homes and independent boarding schools. Also included are provisions restricting the use of wardship by local authorities and various procedural and jurisdictional reforms.

Rules of court and regulations

In addition to the Act's 12 parts there is extensive subordinate legislation with 48 sets of rules and regulations. The rules regulate legal procedures and how the court system works, whilst the regulations specify how the primary legislation must be applied in practice. Both have the same legal effect as the Act and must be complied with.

Guidance documents

Nine volumes of guidance have also been issued (*see* Appendix A). They are not in themselves law but are designed as statements of what is held to be good practice. Their general aim is to explain the Act and give some idea of how it should be implemented. Guidance documents can be quoted or used in court proceedings as well as in local authority policy and practice papers. They could also provide the basis for legal challenge of an authority's action or inaction.
     Other relevant guidance documents are:
The Care of Children: principles and practice in regulations and guidance, HMSO, 1990.
Working Together: a guide to arrangements for inter-agency co-operation for the protection of children from abuse, HMSO, 1991.
Protecting Children: a guide for social workers undertaking a comprehensive assessment, HMSO, 1991.

Aims and objectives of the Act

The main aims are to:

1. Consolidate private and public law

Until the Children Act was passed the development of childcare law had been sporadic and fragmented. It was contained in a huge volume of different statutes and judicial decisions, many of which had been enacted in response to a particular crisis rather than as a coherent element in a general strategy. This unwieldy mass is now replaced by one single, comprehensive code (nine separate postwar statutes are repealed in full by the Act and many more substantially amended). This brings together almost all the law relating to the care, protection and upbringing of children. This unified approach means that the same terminology and a single court structure apply to both private and public law and also that a consistent set of remedies is available in all courts and proceedings.

2. Reorganize the court system

Important procedural and jurisdictional changes are made to the way courts deal with cases to enable them to take a more proactive supervisory role in proceedings and control how local authorities (likewise lawyers and other professionals) carry out their duties. In addition, a three-tiered court system has been created to ensure that all cases come before the appropriate level of court.

3. Provide new legal remedies to resolve disputes

A range of practical, flexible and interchangeable orders are introduced which are available in all proceedings. This means that a private dispute can be resolved by a public law order and vice versa. The new scheme also aims to widen access to the courts, allowing a greater range of people to initiate proceedings.

4. Encourage new attitudes to the role of the family and the state

Another major aim is to encourage parents and families to take centre stage in children's upbringing. Accordingly, emphasis is placed on support and preventive services with less frequent resort to compulsory measures. This aim has necessitated redefining parental power in terms of parental responsibility and making significant changes to the legal position of those children looked after away from home (reflecting the theme of partnership with parents, children and their families).

5. Realign the balance between children, their parents and the state

Striking a 'better' or 'new' balance between the protection of children, the autonomy and integrity of the family and the role of the state is at the heart of the radical reforms made to the powers of local authorities to intervene in family life. Hence the Act sets a new single standard – based on the concept of 'significant harm' – for compulsory action, and establishes a framework within which social work practice can be made more accountable and consistent. It also seeks to identify and enhance children's legal independence.

6. Introduce new guidelines for court decisions

New principles and concepts are introduced to provide greater coherence to court decisions and encourage greater consistency, clarity and a more systematic approach to decision-making. These emphasize the paramountcy of the child's welfare, the importance of avoiding long, drawn out proceedings and should discourage orders from being made unless they are really necessary.

7. Provide a new regulatory framework for substitute care

A new scheme is created to monitor and control all forms of substitute care. This is intended to develop more confidence in a broad range of services from private homes to day nurseries and child-minders, and to facilitate a 'mixed economy' of service provision.

General principles of the Act

The Act embodies three fundamental principles which are set out in its first Section. These are non-intervention, speedy resolution of disputes and the paramountcy of the child's welfare. Equally important, however, although not made explicit, are another set of related principles which run through the whole Act. These include the belief that the best place for children to be brought up is with their families, the philosophy of partnership and the legal recognition of children's independent rights.

The child's welfare is paramount

Children come first and their welfare (commonly also referred to as their 'best interests') must be the paramount consideration whenever the court makes a decision about their upbringing. This means that although it can take into account all surrounding circumstances, these are only relevant in so far as they cast light on the child's welfare. But although the welfare concept has been a central feature of child law for well over 50 years no statutory attempt has ever been made to clarify its nature or scope, or even to indicate the kinds of factors which courts ought to consider.

Not surprisingly, therefore, and especially since it is such an indeterminate concept, the courts had very wide discretion in deciding what they thought was best for a child. Decisions were frequently inconsistent, arbitrary and rarely predictable. In one recent case, for example, an unemployed father, who had been successfully looking after his child, lost custody because it 'was his duty to work and support the family' and not stay at home relying upon benefits provided by the welfare state. In another case one of the reasons why a mother – who was a Jehovah's witness – was denied custody of her children was that they would not be able to celebrate Christmas and would therefore be 'deprived of the wholesome joys of life' and 'the charms of crackers and paper hats'.

The 'welfare check list' (Section 1.3)

Although the Act does not define 'welfare', it seeks to improve and standardize the way decisions are made not only by emphasizing the value of welfare reports and the role of guardians ad litem but also by introducing a welfare 'check list'.

This lists the factors the courts must consider in most contested cases and is intended 'to provide greater clarity and consistency and a more systematic approach to decision-making'. The items specified are not in fact new since (with one exception) they repeat concerns which were considered important in previous law and practice.

The value of the check list has yet to be established but in the meantime it should ensure at least that the same basic factors are used by everyone involved in a case. It may also help parents, children and others to understand how decisions are made and enable evidence and other material to be prepared more quickly.

Each factor is considered below.

1. *The ascertainable wishes and feelings of the child concerned (considered in the light of his age and understanding)*

In the past, some courts were willing to listen to children, however their wishes were usually ignored − often because of the belief that they were easily brainwashed or bribed and over-influenced by short-term material gains. Reflecting the influence of the Gillick case, however, the courts are now obliged to consider the child's own wishes and views but are not obliged to follow them. This means that children have a right to be consulted but cannot insist that their views prevail.

According to official guidance, the Act's aim is

> 'to strike a balance between the need to recognise the child as an independent person and to ensure that his views are fully taken into account, and the risk of casting on him the burden of resolving problems caused by his parents or requiring him to choose between them'.

The precise weight to be attached to a child's views will, of course, depend ultimately on the circumstances of each individual case, the nature of the dispute and the age and maturity of the child concerned. But even the views of very young children should not automatically be discounted. In care proceedings and other public law cases, for example, guardians *ad litem* (GALs) attempt to discover the views of children as young as three.

2. *His physical, emotional and educational needs*

The concept of 'need' is very broad and can include a wide variety of considerations. It is also a relative term as different children will have different needs depending on their own circumstances. Nevertheless, the intention is that as far as possible an objective assessment should be made. Hence a child's physical needs are likely to include adequate day-to-day care such as housing, food and clothing. Any special health care needs must also be met. So if, for example, a child requires regular medical treatment, the availability of appropriate local facilities will clearly be an important or even decisive factor.

Emotional needs, although less determinate, are likely to include 'love, care, and emotional support'. In particular, past cases suggest that the courts are especially concerned to respect and sustain existing attachments and to maintain continuity of care and the child's ties with members of his or her family.

Educational needs are often confined to questions of schooling but can also include education in the broader sense and what the child does after school. This means that 'education' can cover virtually anything to do with upbringing, possibly even an assessment of parental attitudes to discipline. Finally, any special educational needs will also have to be considered.

3. The likely effect of any change in circumstances

A number of studies have highlighted how preserving the status quo is extremely important in determining a child's adjustment to family breakdown. Children need consistency and stability in their relationships and environment. If existing arrangements are well-established and successful the courts are unlikely to change them.

4. His age, sex, background and any personal characteristic which the court considers relevant

Age is clearly a significant factor in assessing a child's physical, emotional and educational needs. It is also linked with other factors such as a child's wishes and feelings. Sex could be important, most notably in residential disputes when a parent of the same sex may be better able to understand and deal with the various physical and emotional needs and problems of the child as he or she grows up. Background can mean almost anything. It could include family environment, in which case courts should take into account ethnic, racial, cultural and linguistic factors. Religious upbringing might also be significant, especially if there is concern about any social limitations which may be imposed on a child's activities by parents' adherence to a particular sect. Characteristic is also a broad term covering physical and emotional factors. A child might, for example, have a disability or chronic illness, or perhaps special educational needs.

5. Any harm which he has suffered or is at risk of suffering

This concept covers ill treatment and the impairment of health or development – both physical and psychological. It covers past 'harm' as well as that which may occur in the future.

6. How capable each of his parents (or any other person in relation to whom the court considers the question to be relevant) is of meeting his needs

'Capability' in this context covers the abilities of parents and other carers to provide for a child's emotional, physical and educational needs. In assessing this the court will take behaviour or lifestyle into account in so far as it has a direct bearing on the child's welfare. If the parents are not full-time carers the court will have to be satisfied of the capabilities of other potential carers, such as new partners, step-parents or grandparents. Child care arrangements outside the family, including child-minders and nurseries, may also need to be assessed.

7. *The range of powers available to the court under this Act in the proceedings in question*

This part of the check list is new. It reminds the court that it has wide powers under the Act and can select any appropriate remedy from the full list of orders available. So the court is not restricted to considering just the one order which is being sought. It can instead, substitute another one. It can also mix and match orders, for example, by ordering that a child live with one parent but, at the same time, be supervised by the local authority.

When must the check list be considered?

The check list must be applied by a court when it is considering the making, variation, or discharge of a Section 8 order which is opposed (this will usually involve private law disputes). It must also be applied in Part IV public law proceedings, ie care, supervision, care contact or education supervision orders.

Welfare reports

A court's power to order welfare reports has been extended by the Act. They can now be obtained in any question with respect to a child. The welfare officer's task is to prepare a report about the child's and family's environment and its preparation will invariably involve visits to the child's home and interviews with the child, his or her parents and anyone else who may have relevant information, for example, teachers and relatives. Welfare reports are confidential but can be inspected by the parties and their advisers. They usually contain a recommendation to the court which it is not obliged to follow.

Non-intervention (Section 1(5))

The Act introduces a new 'non-intervention' or 'minimum intervention' principle which is that the court should not make an order 'unless it considers that doing so would be better for the child than making no order at all'. This phrase effectively creates a presumption against court action unless it is absolutely necessary and will positively improve the child's welfare. This principle has been described as a 'key to an understanding of the whole Act' and an explicit attempt to 'privatize' and 'deregulate' the family by minimizing the role of the state. Whilst these interpretations are debatable the principle undoubtedly reflects the Act's fundamental philosophy 'that children are best cared for within the family with both parents playing a full part and without resort to legal proceedings' (Introduction to the Children Act, HMSO, 1989, para 1.3).

The presumption against intervention has important implications for both private and public law proceedings. In private disputes such as divorce it is intended to discourage orders being routinely made as part of the 'divorce package' when there is no need for them. By restricting orders to cases where there is a demonstrable need, parental agreement and co-operation is expected to be encouraged.

In public proceedings non-intervention means that the court is not bound to make an order just because the relevant criteria have been met. In the past there was some concern that once the grounds for making an order were made out, then it was made irrespective of whether it would or even could benefit the child. But now the court must ask itself: is the order going to promote the child's welfare or are other arrangements preferable; for example, the provision of voluntary support or preventive services?

Less delay (Section 1(2))

This principle creates a presumption that delay in settling disputes about children is harmful and should, if possible, be avoided. This 'no-delay' or 'no-drift' principle is supplemented by various other provisions, for example, the court can draw up timetables and give directions to speed up proceedings. The reason for this new approach is the belief that a 'child's sense of time may be more acute than an adult's and that protracted proceedings are deeply damaging, not only because of the uncertainty they bring a child, but also because of the harm they do to the parents' relationship and their capacity to co-operate with each other in the future'.

It should be noted that the assumption that delay is harmful is only a general statement of principle. There may well be instances when delay could be beneficial, perhaps because more time is needed to assess a child, prepare a welfare report, allow things to settle down or for conciliation.

Children and their families

As noted earlier the Act rests on the belief that the best place for children to grow up is with their families. Parents are usually, therefore, the primary agents of their children's welfare. Although the non-intervention principle is the most explicit statement of this belief it is also reflected in a number of other provisions, notably the new concept of 'parental responsibility' and the increased emphasis on the provision of services to children 'in need'. In addition, where children are living away from home, there are provisions aimed at maintaining their links with familiar people and places and promoting reunification and rehabilitation.

Partnership and co-operation

A key theme in the Act is that of partnership between local authorities, parents and children. The concept of partnership is not new, but is based on well-established beliefs and practices. It applies when children are being supported at home as well as when they are being looked after elsewhere. It involves keeping parents and children fully informed, consulting them and strengthening their rights to challenge decisions. For the first time, too, specific reference is made in the Act to race, culture and language as factors to be considered in making decisions about a child's care. Partnership between local authority social services departments, other local authority departments (eg housing and health), the voluntary and independent sector and other agencies is also intended so that a 'seamless service' can be provided.

The child's voice

The Act attempts to identify the independent rights of children and enhance their legal status. They are, for example, (providing they have reached the required level of understanding) given the right to refuse medical and psychiatric examinations and assessments in various public law contexts and to initiate court proceedings. In certain circumstances too, they can refer themselves into local authority accommodation and decide when to leave. They must also be consulted about decisions which affect them. In addition, their wishes head the welfare 'check list'.

2

Legal Parentage and Parental Responsibility

This chapter is divided into two sections. The first will focus on establishing who in law is regarded as a parent, ie determining legal parentage. The second will define the scope and nature of parental responsibility.

Legal parentage: who is a parent?

Determining legal parentage is important for three main reasons. First, legislation (which may either create rights or impose duties) frequently refers to a child's 'parents'. Without clear guidelines this is a title which could be claimed by any one of the following three categories.

- *Genetic parents*: those who have provided the genetic material resulting in the child's conception
- *Social parents*: those with no biological or genetic link with the child but who are actually caring for it or who intend to do so, for example foster parents, relatives or commissioning 'parents' in a surrogacy arrangement (*see* below)
- A *'carrying' parent*: the woman who carries and gives birth to a child but who may not have provided any of its genetic make-up (some or all of which has been provided by another couple).

Secondly, determining who the law regards as a child's legal parents will assist in deciding who has parental responsibility under the Children Act and liability to support the child under, for example, the Child Support Act 1991.

The third reason for establishing legal parentage is that it may arise in disputes about inheritance rights, succession to property and immigration status.

In the past the determination of parenthood was relatively straightforward. But recent developments, notably, advances in reproductive technology and 'scientific testing', have raised fundamental questions about legal parentage and made it increasingly difficult to establish who is a child's legal mother and father. As the following techniques commonly used in human assisted reproduction demonstrate, it is now possible for a child to be born to parents who are neither genetically nor socially linked to it.

AID (Artificial Insemination by a Donor)

This technique involves artificially inseminating a woman with sperm obtained from a donor. If married or co-habiting couples use this method and the donated sperm is the husband's or partner's the child's genetic and legal parentage coincide. But if the donated sperm is neither the husband's nor partner's, questions will arise as to whether the donor – who is undoubtedly the genetic father – should be regarded as the child's legal father.

IVF (In Vitro Fertilization)

This entails fertilizing an egg outside the body. The embryo is then transferred back into the woman's womb. This technique can take different forms. Traditionally, it involves sperm donated by the husband or partner of the woman, in which case the child is genetically related to both its parents. But if donated sperm or ova or both are used, the child may be genetically related to only one of its parents or possibly neither.

GIFT (Gamete Intrafallopian Transfer)

This relatively new technique involves transferring ova, sperm or both directly into the woman's Fallopian tubes so that fertilization can occur *in vivo* (in the womb). If it involves donated gametes the child is again not genetically related to either of its parents.

Surrogacy

This is an arrangement in which one woman carries a child for another with the intention that the child should be handed over after the birth to the 'commissioning parents'. There are various different types of arrangements which are now regulated by the Surrogacy Arrangements Act 1985. The most usual is 'partial surrogacy' which involves insemination of the surrogate with the commissioning father's sperm. Alternatively 'full or total surrogacy' (also called womb-leasing) can be arranged, whereby the commissioning woman provides the ovum which is fertilized *in vitro* or *in vivo* with her husband's or partner's sperm. In this instance the carrying woman is not genetically related to the child she carries.

Effect of Human Fertilization and Embryology Act 1990

Because of the increasing use of these techniques and the inability of the existing legal framework to accommodate them, the Human Fertilization and Embryology Act 1990 introduced new rules about legal parentage and clarified the legal status of a child born as a result of egg donation or embryo transfer.

In summary, these rules provide that 'the woman who is carrying or has carried a child as a result of the placing in her of an embryo or of sperm and eggs is to be treated as the mother'. This makes it clear that a child's legal mother is the woman who carries and gives birth to it, regardless of its genetic mother.

Implicitly it also means that a woman is regarded as a legal mother if she gives birth to a child to whom she is the genetic mother.

The definition of 'father' in the Act is complex but basically it provides that generally the legal father of a child is the person who provides the sperm which results in conception. This basic rule is subject to two exceptions. The first covers married couples and provides that if the wife has a child following treatment (for example embryo transfer, GIFT, artificial insemination) then it is the husband rather than the sperm donor who is the legal father. This is the case unless he can show he did not consent to the treatment and can rebut the presumption that a mother's husband is the father of any child she bears.

The second exception covers unmarried couples and provides that where donated sperm is used for a woman in the course of treatment provided under the licensing procedure of the Act, the woman's partner – not the sperm donor – is the legal father of the child. In other words an unmarried partner can acquire the legal status of father of his partner's child even though he is not the genetic father.

In both these exceptions it is the clear policy of the Act to prevent the sperm donor from being treated as the legal father.

Proving parenthood

Even though the Human Fertilization and Embryology Act 1990 clarifies legal parenthood, disputes may still arise. For example, a man may deny paternity to avoid paying child maintenance. In such cases parentage may need to be proved. This can be done either by obtaining a declaration of parentage from a court or in the following ways.

Birth registration

The birth of every child must be registered within 42 days. Birth registration is the most usual method of establishing legal parentage and the entry of a man's name as a child's father can be crucial evidence of paternity. If the parents are married either the husband or wife can register the husband's name as the father. But the rights of an unmarried father to register his name are more limited and only apply if certain conditions are met.

Blood tests and scientific evidence

Two tests are currently available. Blood tests are the more traditional and cheapest type but they are only exclusionary. This means they can eliminate the possibility that a person is a child's parent, but they can never directly and conclusively prove he or she is the parent. More recent scientific tests, notably DNA fingerprinting, are more sophisticated and accurate and can provide positive proof of parentage.

Parental responsibility

'Parental responsibility' is the new term used in the Act to describe the legal authority parents have over their children. It replaces the phrase 'parental rights' which has long been thought inappropriate largely because of its proprietorial connotations. It is intended to reinforce the idea that the law gives parents authority to make decisions about their children's lives, not as a reward of parenthood but so that they can fulfil their role as parents and 'raise their child to become a properly developed adult both physically and morally'. The new vocabulary is also intended to emphasize that responsibility for children belongs to their parents, not the state.

But what is the scope and nature of parental responsibility? What does it actually entitle a parent to do? Unfortunately the Act provides very little guidance on this. It simply says that the new concept means

> 'all the rights, duties, powers, responsibilities and authority which by law a parent of a child has in relation to the child and his property' (Section 3(1)).

The Act, therefore, does not contain a comprehensive definition of parental responsibility nor does it provide a list of the things parents can or cannot do. Moreover it does not even alter the extent or scope of the authority parents had before the Children Act came into force. Essentially the new vocabulary is a shorthand expression of symbolic importance in that it might encourage a change in perception of the parental role. It is useful, too, since it is consistently used to describe how people other than parents are entitled to exercise authority – a reform which does much to clarify their legal position.

Scope of parental responsibility

To find out what comprises parental responsibility it is therefore necessary to go outside the Act and, although there is no agreed list of actions, those with responsibility can take the following is a description of those most commonly accepted.

1. Providing a home (sometimes called 'physical possession')

This is perhaps one of the most important aspects of parental responsibility since it involves caring for and bringing up a child. Having the right to care for a child means deciding how to meet his or her physical needs, including food, shelter, clothing and hygiene, and emotional needs. Put very broadly it involves determining how and where a child spends its time. It thus includes making major decisions such as where and with whom a child should live as well as more mundane decisions, for example what a child should eat or wear.

The right to care for a child is protected by the criminal law and there are a number of offences, such as kidnapping and child abduction, which can be committed if children are removed without lawful authority.

2. Contact

For parents who are not living with their children the right to have contact with them is especially important. The word 'contact' replaces the term 'access' but its scope is just as broad. It is not confined just to face-to-face physical contact but can also cover contact in the form of letters and telephone calls. Although it is generally assumed that children benefit from contact with their parents it is not an absolute right. Accordingly there may well be occasions when contact may be restricted or prevented, for example in cases of sexual abuse.

3. Discipline

A person with parental responsibility can lawfully discipline a child by using corporal punishment. Corporal punishment means any intentional application of force and includes slapping, smacking, hitting with implements, throwing missiles and rough handling. But it must be 'moderate' and 'reasonable', ie appropriate to the child's age, health, physique, understanding and strength. Discipline or punishment which fails to conform to this standard – imprecise though it may be – can result in criminal or civil proceedings.

A person *in loco parentis* ie someone who has been entrusted with the child's care, also has the power to discipline and punish. Corporal punishment is, however, now banned in most schools (state, grant maintained and some, but not all, independent schools), community homes, secure units, voluntary homes, registered children's homes, residential care homes and state foster placements (*see* detailed regulations on disciplinary measures in Guidance Volume 4, Annex A).

4. Religious upbringing

Parents have the right to decide what religious faith their child should follow if any. The Education Act 1988 also gives them the right to exclude their child from religious study lessons and school assembly. Parental choice of religion will not, however, prevail over the views of a 'mature' child who understands the implications of his or her decision. Nor will a child be obliged to follow a religion which is 'harmful'. It is also worth noting that when children are being looked after by a local authority it must take positive steps to ensure that they can practise their religion. Similarly, adoption agencies must have regard to a child's religion when arranging a placement.

5. Name

It is usual, but not obligatory, for a child of married parents to take the father's surname. Neither parent can then change it without the other's consent or a court order. But if both parents agree the child's surname can be easily changed either informally or formally.

Children of unmarried parents usually take their mother's surname, but again this is just convention and there is no legal reason why the father's surname should not be used. There are also various, fairly complex provisions, regulating the entry of the unmarried father's name on the birth certificate.

When a child is in care a local authority cannot change his or her surname without the written consent of every person with parental responsibility or the court's permission.

6. Education

Parents have a wide discretion in deciding how their children should be educated, although they are legally obliged to ensure that those of compulsory school age (between five and 16) receive sufficient full-time education suitable to their age, aptitude, ability and any special educational needs they may have. Usually children go to school (state or private) but parents can opt out of the school system altogether – with local authority approval – by providing 'alternative' appropriate education at home.

Recent legislation, notably the Education Act 1980, has attempted to give parents more influence over their child's education. In particular they now have the right to express a preference for a particular school, which education authorities must comply with (although this is not an absolute duty). Parents are also entitled to receive much more information about schools such as their examination results and curriculum.

Failure to ensure that a child is educated can result in criminal liability. An education supervision order may also be made (*see* Chapter 7) which gives a 'supervisor' wide powers to control the child's education.

The law on children with 'special educational needs' is mainly contained in the Education Act 1981. It provides a structure whereby local education authorities (LEAs), parents and schools can co-operate in identifying, assessing and meeting any special needs (*see* Chapter 11).

The education of a child in local authority care is governed by regulations (*see* Guidance Volume 4, Annex A).

7. Marriage

A child under 16 cannot get married. If the child is 16 but under 18 (and not a widow or widower) parental consent is necessary, usually from both parents. If parental consent is unobtainable the marriage can still take place as a court may authorize it instead. Other consents may also be necessary such as from the local authority if the child is subject to a care order.

8. Travel and emigration

Parental consent is required before a passport will be issued to a child under 18 (other than a one year British visitor's passport). Those under 16 can be included in their parents' passport. Furthermore any person with parental responsibility may ask the United Kingdom passport agency not to issue a passport allowing the child to go abroad without the knowledge of that person. Other measures can also be taken to prevent a child being abducted (under the Child Abduction Act 1984). There are also restrictions on taking a child abroad when a care order or residence order is in force. These are fairly complex but their broad effect is that anyone with parental responsibility must consent to the child going abroad for more than one month. On the other hand those with sole parental responsibility or with joint parental responsibility can agree to arrange for the child's removal from the United Kingdom for any period.

9. Consent to medical treatment

This is covered in Chapter 3.

10. Miscellaneous powers

Other actions which can be taken by those with parental responsibility include the right to act on the child's behalf in legal proceedings providing there is no conflict of interest; to appoint a guardian; to consent to adoption; to administer the child's property and inherit it on intestacy.

Finally something must be said about the various 'duties' which are conventionally held to be part of parental responsibility, although again their scope and extent have never been statutorily listed. There are three general duties: to maintain, to educate and to protect children from 'physical and moral harm'. Protection from physical harm involves providing the 'necessities of life' such as food, shelter, clothing and medical aid. Whilst 'moral' protection aims to protect the child's character and moral upbringing. Predictably there is extensive legislation aimed at protecting children from activities deemed inappropriate or dangerous, such as gambling, begging and being tattooed (see also Appendices C and D).

Parents who fail to maintain their children can be compelled to support them and those who abuse or neglect their children may be criminally liable. Compulsory intervention by a local authority might also ensue.

Restrictions on parental responsibility

Although the various aspects of parental responsibility outlined above seem to give parents and others with parental responsibility considerable control over their children's lives, their authority is by no means absolute since it is subject to two major restrictions. The first is the welfare principle. The courts have made it quite clear that parental responsibility must be exercised in accordance with that principle and can be challenged, even overridden if it is not. In other words any dispute about a child's care or upbringing, for example schooling or medical treatment, must be resolved so as to promote and safeguard the child's welfare.

The second limitation derives from the Gillick case which established that 'mature' children can and should have independent control over their own lives in certain circumstances. In considering the extent of parental authority the court stressed that

> 'the legal right of a parent ends at the 18th birthday, and even up till then, it is a dwindling right which the courts will hesitate to enforce against the wishes of the child, the older he is. It starts with a right of control and ends with little more than advice'.

Parental responsibility therefore diminishes as the child matures and gradually acquires sufficient understanding to make his or her own decisions. Furthermore, the Act now requires the child's wishes to be ascertained in most disputes over upbringing (*see* The welfare 'check-list' Section 1(3), Chapter 1).

Who has parental responsibility?

The rules concerning the allocation and acquisition of parental responsibility have been simplified and clarified by the Act. In particular, the position of the unmarried father has been considerably improved. It is also now easier for non-parents such as grandparents or other people to acquire responsibility. The overall effect of the new rules is as follows.

Married parents

If a child is legitimate both parents have automatic parental responsibility. A legitimate child is one whose parents were either married at the time of the child's conception or birth, or who married after that time. This responsibility lasts until a child reaches 18 or is adopted and cannot be removed or suspended (although it can be shared) before then whatever type of court order is made. In other words it is unaffected by divorce or separation, although a Section 8 order may limit how it is exercised. Similarly, it is not lost when a local authority acquires parental responsibility as a result of a care order, although its exercise might be limited.

Unmarried parents

When a child's parents are not married only the mother automatically has parental responsibility. Again this only ceases when the child is adopted or reaches 18. An unmarried father does not automatically have parental responsibility, even if he is maintaining or living with his child's mother, but can acquire it by:

- marrying the mother or adopting his child
- obtaining a court order (ie a parental responsibility or residence order)
- being appointed a guardian
- making a parental responsibility agreement with the mother.

The parental responsibility agreement is a new, simple and cheap procedure introduced by the Act. It involves signing a prescribed form (costing £1) which then has to be officially recorded.

Both parental responsibility orders and agreements can be brought to an end by the court on application by any person with parental responsibility for the child, or the child, provided he or she has the court's leave and sufficient understanding to make the application.

Other people

Other people, for example relatives and step-parents, can also acquire parental responsibility as a result of:

- a residence order
- adoption
- being appointed a guardian
- an emergency protection order.

In addition local authorities also acquire parental responsibility when a care order and emergency protection order is in force. But a court order is necessary for this to happen unlike the previous law when parental rights could be transferred by a very unpopular and controversial administrative procedure.

However, the parental responsibility acquired by non-parents is less enduring and less extensive than that of parents. It does not, for example, include the right to consent to adoption or appoint a guardian. Furthermore it can lapse automatically such as when the residence order or care order ends.

Sharing parental responsibility

Because the Act implicitly provides that a person with responsibility does not lose it just because someone else subsequently also acquires it (Section 2(6)) there may be instances where parental responsibility will be held simultaneously. In other words it will be shared by – or divided between – different people at the same time. For example, by grandparents and the child's mother or by the local authority and the child's parents.

What does sharing responsibility mean in practice? Does each person with parental responsibility have to consult everyone else with responsibility before making a decision about the child or can each one act independently? In private law disputes, such as divorce, sharing responsibility in theory means that both parents (and anyone else who is sharing responsibility with them, for example a grandmother in whose favour there is a residence order) have the right to take decisions about the child's upbringing. In practice, of course, it is the person actually caring for the child on a day-to-day basis who will have most control over the child's movements. Note also, that if a child's parents are not married the father will only retain responsibility if he has acquired it before the separation.

Furthermore, the Act allows everyone with parental responsibility to act alone (subject to any restriction imposed by a court order) when exercising their responsibility. There is no duty to consult anyone else with parental responsibility before acting. This means disputes will have to be resolved either by negotiation or court proceedings.

When a care order or emergency protection order is made parental authority is again shared, usually by the child's parents and the local authority. A local authority can, however, limit and control the way parents exercise their responsibility, a power it is expected to use sparingly and only when necessary to promote and safeguard the child's welfare.

Delegation of parental responsibility

A person with parental responsibility cannot surrender or transfer it but he or she can arrange for particular aspects of it to be taken over by someone else (Section 3(5)). For example, a trip abroad or stay in hospital may necessitate a temporary arrangement. In these situations the person who is looking after the child does not have parental responsibility but does have the right to 'do what is reasonable in all the circumstances of the case for the purpose of safeguarding or promoting the child's welfare'. The scope of this authority is uncertain but it would probably permit the temporary carer to arrange urgent medical treatment.

Case studies

Case study 1

Ann, a lively seven-year-old, falls off a swing in the school playground. At first it seems no more than a minor accident but by lunchtime she is looking very pale and says she feels sick. As Ann's parents are on a touring holiday abroad the school telephones her Aunt, Betty, who is looking after her, to take her home. Betty takes Ann straight to the local hospital. The casualty officer considers medical treatment to be necessary.

1. Who has parental responsibility for Ann and therefore the right to consent to medical treatment on her behalf?
2. What difference would it make if Ann's parents were not married?
3. Who can authorize treatment if no-one with parental responsibility can be contacted?
4. If no-one is available to give consent (or consent is refused) could hospital staff authorize treatment?
5. At what age could Ann herself give consent to treatment?

Solutions

1. As Ann's parents are married they both automatically have parental responsibility for her and therefore the independent right to consent to medical treatment on her behalf.

2. If Ann's parents were not married then only her mother would automatically have parental responsibility and her father would need to have acquired parental responsibility (ie by making a parental responsibility agreement with the mother) before he could give consent to treatment.

3. Ann's current carer Betty would have the right to authorize treatment by virtue of Section 3(5) of the Children Act which gives temporary carers the right to 'do what is reasonable in all the circumstances of the case for the purpose of safeguarding or promoting the child's welfare'. Note, however, that if treatment was not urgently required it should be postponed until Ann's parents return home and give their consent.

4. If Betty refused to give consent or despite currently caring for Ann could not be contacted then hospital staff could treat Ann without obtaining anyone's consent. They could only act under their own authority, however, if emergency treatment was necessary to safeguard Ann's life. In less urgent cases they should not act until someone with parental responsibility gives consent or if this is refused until court proceedings (ie a specific issue order) has resolved the matter.

5. Ann's right to consent depends on whether she is considered 'Gillick competent' which is a matter of individual professional judgement. This means she must have reached a sufficient age and understanding to take her own informed medical decision. But, given Ann's young age, it is unlikely that she would be considered old enough to consent herself.

Case study 2

Barry is 14 and has been in the care of the local authority for the past year. His father died several months before the care order was made and his mother, Christina, was unable to look after him due to a long-term drinking problem. For the first few months Barry was in care, Christina visited him quite regularly at the home of his foster parents Mr and Mrs Chowdry. For the last three months though, Christina has not been in touch at all because she has been in and out of hospital due to a rapid deterioration in her mental health.

Last night Barry accidentally fell down the stairs and broke his leg in several places. He is rushed to hospital where Mr and Mrs Chowdry are told that surgery is necessary. They tell hospital staff that unfortunately Christina is unable to give consent at the moment and is unlikely to be in a fit state to do so for several weeks.

1. Who can consent to surgery for Barry?
2. Can Barry himself give consent to surgery?
3. As local authority foster parents what rights do Mr and Mrs Chowdry have to give consent?

Solutions

1. The local authority has parental responsibility as a result of the care order. They share this responsibility with Christina but since the Children Act provides that when more than one person has such responsibility each can act alone in meeting that

responsibility, the local authority's sole consent is sufficient for surgery to be carried out.

2. If Barry is considered sufficiently mature to make an informed decision about his medical care (ie he passes the 'Gillick' test) then he himself can consent to treatment.

3. If urgent surgery is required and the local authority cannot be contacted in time then either Mr or Mrs Chowdry as temporary carers could consent under Section 3(5) of the Children Act (*see* Case study 1 (3) above).

Case study 3

Cherry is five months old and lives with her parents, Donna and Eric (who are not married) and twin five-year-old brothers. The family live in very damp, crowded accommodation and the children often have bad coughs and colds lasting several weeks. In fact Cherry herself had a serious chest infection soon after she was born but she is now much better and due to be immunized. When Donna takes her to the health centre however, Eric rushes in and says that Cherry cannot be immunized because he has arranged for a course of homoeopathic treatment and has an appointment with the homoeopath the following morning. The health visitor is very anxious that Cherry should be immunized as soon as possible because there is an outbreak of whooping cough on the estate where the family live.

1. Who has the right to consent to Cherry's immunization?
2. Has Eric the right to prevent it?
3. How can Eric control Cherry's medical treatment?
4. If Eric does acquire parental responsibility and he and Donna disagree about immunization, can Cherry still be immunized?

Solutions

1. Since Cherry's parents are not married only Donna has automatic parental responsibility and the right to consent to Cherry being immunized.

2. Unless Eric has acquired parental responsibility (*see* (3) below) he has no right to consent to, or refuse, permission for immunization. He could, however, apply for a prohibited steps order to prevent treatment.

3. Apart from applying for a prohibited steps order to prevent treatment Eric could acquire parental responsibility, for example by applying for a parental responsibility order. This would then give him an independent right to consent to or refuse medical treatment for Cherry.

4. If Eric does have parental responsibility he will share it with Donna and Cherry's immunization should be postponed until their disagreement is resolved. Eric could apply for a prohibited steps order to prevent the immunization and Donna would seek a specific issue order to permit it.

3

Consent to Treatment

The right to consent to medical treatment on behalf of a child is an aspect of parental responsibility which has long been controversial. Although it was perhaps the Gillick case in 1986 which first catapulted the issue into public debate, a number of other highly publicized health-related disputes in the last decade have also centred on consent. For example, whether a mature 12-year-old can consent to an abortion despite parental opposition or when treatment for a seriously ill new-born baby can be undertaken against parents' wishes. Similarly, the question of consent is also central in certain treatment for mentally handicapped minors, such as sterilization. To understand how these kinds of disputes are resolved, however, the basic legal principles relating to consent need to be outlined.

Basic principles

Except in special circumstances (*see* below) every mentally competent adult patient has an absolute legal right to give or withhold consent to medical treatment or examination. This means that subject to certain exceptions health professionals must not do anything to a patient unless they have first obtained the patient's agreement. To be legally valid though, such consent must fulfil certain criteria. In summary they are as follows.

Consent must be effectively obtained

The law does not lay down any specific rules about the form of consent which can be expressed (either oral or written) or implied. In practice, express written consent is obtained for any procedure or treatment carrying any substantial risks or side-effects (ie general anaesthesia, surgery, certain forms of drug therapy). The main purpose of written consent is that it provides the best evidence or 'proof' that consent was actually sought and obtained. However a patient's signature on the consent form is not proof itself and may well be worthless if he or she was not given appropriate information or was incapable of understanding the significance of signing the form (*see* below).

For 'less risky' procedures such as blood tests and other similar routine procedures express oral consent may be sufficient. In many cases, however, patients do not give their express consent in clear and explicit terms, either orally or in writing. Nevertheless their agreement can be implied from their actions. Examples of such 'implied' consent are again common and nurses typically rely on it for nursing care when, for example, patients roll up their sleeves for an injection or open their mouths for an examination. In situations like these consent can be implied from the circumstances, even though care should always be taken to ensure that the patient is actually agreeing. Silence cannot be assumed to be consent.

Consent must be voluntary

Consent must be voluntary and not obtained by coercion, manipulation, duress or undue influence. In Re T (Adult: Refusal of Treatment (1992) 3 WLR 782) for example, the court overrode the refusal of consent to a blood transfusion by a 20-year-old pregnant woman. Before losing consciousness she had expressly refused a transfusion on religious grounds but the court held that this refusal was limited in scope because of the undue pressure and influence exerted by her mother (a Jehovah's Witness). In these circumstances her refusal did not represent her own independent decision and it was therefore lawful for the hospital to administer blood to her if it was in her best interests.

Patients must be mentally competent

For consent or refusal to be valid patients must be mentally competent, ie they must have the capacity to understand what is being proposed and the nature of the choice they are making. But what is the test for competency? Given that the degree of competency required will vary according to the complexity of the issues involved, the law does not lay down any rigid criteria or single test for competency. Nevertheless it has been suggested that at least five criteria can be used to decide whether a patient understands proposed treatment:

- evidencing of choice
- reasonable outcome of choice
- choice based on rational reasons
- ability to understand and actual understanding.

Competency can be affected by both long-term and short-term factors. In some cases, for example, incompetency may be caused by mental illness or retarded development. In other cases temporary factors such as unconsciousness, confusion or the effects of fatigue, drugs, pain or shock may have affected capacity.

What information must patients be given?

It has long been established that consent can only be valid if patients have been told in broad terms about the nature and effects of the proposed procedures. This does not mean that patients are entitled to know everything, although lack of certain information may give rise to legal action (*see* below). Nevertheless they are expected to be well-informed and not misled. They must be given sufficient accurate information about the purpose, nature, likely effects and risks of treatment, including the likelihood of its success and possible alternatives, in order to make a valid decision.

Exceptions to the principle of consent

The following are examples of when examination or treatment can be carried out without the patient's consent.

- Emergencies where the patient is unconscious (and has not previously indicated his or her wishes) and treatment is necessary to save life, or a condition is discovered which it would be unreasonable to postpone treating. However, the treatment must be limited to that which is necessary to safeguard the life and health of the patient.
- Where legislation (ie Public Health (Control of Disease) Act 1984) provides for compulsory examination.
- Where detention and treatment for mental disorder is authorized under the Mental Health Act 1983.
- Where the patient is incapable of giving consent by reason of mental disorder and the treatment is 'in the patient's best interests', ie it is necessary to preserve life, health or well-being, and practitioners act in accordance with a practice accepted at the time by a responsible body of medical opinion skilled in the particular form of treatment in question.

Furthermore, according to Re F (1989) 2 WLR 1025, if certain forms of treatment in the so-called 'special category' (ie sterilization to prevent pregnancy and *inter vivos* organ donation for transplant) are proposed in respect of an adult who is incompetent then, as a matter of good practice, a declaration should be sought from a court as to whether the proposed treatment is lawful (ie is in the patient's best interests). The court's assistance can also be sought in other cases, especially in life-threatening situations where there is doubt as to the validity of a refusal to consent.

- In certain cases involving children (*see* below).

For further guidance on basic principles of consent and consent forms *see NHS Management Executive: A guide to consent for examination or treatment*, Health Circular HC(90)22.

Acting without consent

Except in the circumstances mentioned above non-consensual medical procedures (examinations or treatment) may constitute a crime and also give a patient the right to sue for damages in the law of tort. If there is no consent at all, for example because the patient is forcibly treated, then the tort of trespass to the person (also known as battery) is committed. Detention in a hospital or other place without consent could also constitute the tort of false imprisonment. More commonly, however, disputes over consent are likely to be pursued through a negligence action. Here the patient is basically claiming that although he or she gave consent to the procedure the consent is inherently flawed and cannot therefore be regarded as 'real' consent.

The 'flaw' may be that certain risks were not disclosed or the patient was given misleading information. Or perhaps information was not given about alternative treatments or side-effects. In other words there was a breach of duty to inform the patient. But, as was noted above, patients are not legally entitled to know everything about their treatment. They must only be told that which accords with good medical practice or a responsible body of professional opinion. Professionals are thus able to set their own standards of disclosure. In practice, this means that if legal action is taken for withholding information, the case will probably turn on whether the health professional concerned acted in accordance with practice accepted at the time as proper by those skilled in the particular form of treatment in question and if they would have withheld the same information.

Children and consent

Despite a number of recent cases involving children and medical treatment, the law is still in some ways uncertain, especially as regards the rights of young people to refuse examinations and assessment under the Children Act. The precise legal parameters of the Gillick case also remain unclear. Does it give young people the right to refuse treatment, for example, and what degree of understanding must a child achieve to be considered 'Gillick competent'? Bearing in mind these uncertainties the present state of the law is as follows.

Sixteen- and seventeen-year-olds

General provisions

According to Section 8 of the Family Law Reform Act 1969 competent young people over the age of 16 can give valid consent to any surgical, medical or dental treatment without regard to their parents' wishes. In this context treatment includes any procedure undertaken for the purposes of diagnosis and procedures, such as the administration of anaesthetics which are ancillary to treatment. This provision also implicitly includes examinations and assessments but not the donation of organs or blood (blood donation by 16-year-olds would nevertheless be covered by the common law).

At 16 people can choose their own doctor and can also seek informal admission to a hospital or mental nursing home under the Mental Health Act 1983 (Section 131).

Although competent minors of 16 and 17 can give such consent as if they were adults they do not have complete autonomy. This is because it now seems that their consent can be overridden by a court (*see* Re W, below). The consent of a competent 16- or 17-year-old cannot, however, be overridden by a person with parental responsibility.

People of 16 and 17 only achieve adult status if they are mentally competent. If they are not competent because of mental illness or another disability (*see* above for assessment of competence) then anyone with parental responsibility, likewise a court, can consent on their behalf. If more than one person has parental responsibility for a child, each one of them may act alone and give consent without the other or others' in meeting that responsibility (Children Act, Section 2(7)).

Various provisions of the Mental Health Act 1983 also apply to people of 16 and 17. This means they will be subject to the same mental health provisions and safeguards as an adult. Additionally, if they are incapable of making their own decisions then again anyone with parental responsibility can arrange for their informal admission to hospital for treatment of mental disorder.

Refusing consent

Until recently it was assumed that competent people of 16 and 17 had the right to refuse treatment. But the recent case of Re W (a minor) (medical treatment) (1992) 3 WLR 758 seems to suggest otherwise, at least in respect of life-threatening situations. The case concerned a 16-year-old anorexic girl in care of the local authority who was refusing to be treated. When the case was heard her weight was down to 35 kg (her height was 1.7 metres) and she had not taken any solid food for the previous seven days. Medical opinion was unanimous that should she continue in this way, within a week her capacity to have children would be seriously at risk and a little later her life might also be in danger. Given these circumstances and the fact that anorexia was said to be capable of destroying the ability to make an informed choice, the court concluded the following.

1. That even when a person has reached 16, if they refused consent then anyone with parental responsibility could override their refusal and give consent (irrespective of the minor's competence) on their behalf until the age of 18.
2. Similarly, the court has a right to override their refusal and authorize treatment, again irrespective of the minor's competence.
3. It is important in evaluating the capacity of a young person to consent, to take into account the impact of any illness or condition which is being treated.
4. A young person's refusal is a very important consideration – and increasingly so with their greater age and maturity – in making clinical judgements (likewise for those with parental responsibility and the courts in deciding themselves to give consent).

Unsurprisingly perhaps the court's decision was controversial, not just because it significantly eroded the autonomy of mature young people to take their own medical decisions but also because it has left the law in an uncertain state. Does it, for example, only give the courts and those with parental responsibility the right to override refusal in cases where a young person's life is in danger? Or does it extend beyond that to non-life saving, but nevertheless controversial or disputed, treatment? Furthermore, the relevance of the Mental Health Act 1983 does not appear to have been fully considered: Should a young person come within the definitions found there before his or her refusal is overruled?

Children under sixteen: 'Gillick competent'

The rights of minors under 16 to make independent medical decisions were established in the landmark Gillick case which gave rise to the phrase 'Gillick competent'. In the case Mrs Gillick claimed that a circular issued by the DHSS advising doctors that they could give contraceptive treatment to girls under 16 without their parents' knowledge or consent, was unlawful. Her claim failed because the court refused to recognize the concept of absolute parental authority. A parent's powers of control were said to 'dwindle as a child grew older and developed the capacity for independent decision-making'. Accordingly, girls under 16 could consent to contraceptive treatment without obtaining parental approval provided they were sufficiently mature, both emotionally and intellectually, to understand its nature and implications.

Although the Gillick case specifically dealt with contraception, the concept of Gillick competence has been applied to other types of medical care involving children under 16 (see Re R and Re E below). But what precisely does the phrase 'Gillick competent' mean? Although commonly used in practice for nearly a decade it is still a subject of debate. Neither is it clear as to when a child should, or should not, be considered competent.

Assessing Gillick competence

Whether a child has sufficient maturity, understanding and intelligence to consent to what is proposed is ultimately a question of fact. Capacity is, however, clearly not automatically acquired at a fixed age, although the ability to understand will normally increase with age. Moreover, the degree of understanding and intelligence required inevitably varies according to the complexity of the issues involved. In other words the degree of understanding increases with the complexity of the proposed treatment. Some decisions, such as contraceptive treatment, may, therefore, require a very high level of understanding and intelligence, whereas others, such as minor dental treatment may require a much less developed intellectual maturity.

It also now seems to have been established, following Re R (a minor) (Wardship: medical treatment) (1991) 4 All ER 177 that Gillick competence is a developmental concept. As such it must be assessed on a broad, long-term basis, taking into account a child's whole medical history and background, as distinct from a 'snap-shot' approach. This means that – in relation to a child with a mental disability – the child is not Gillick competent if his or her capacity to make informed decisions fluctuates.

Re R concerned a girl who was nearly 16. She suffered from a cyclical mental illness with paranoid and psychotic phases during which her behaviour was aggressive, violent and suicidal. During the less acute phases of her illness she was sufficiently rational to give valid consent to treatment, including sedation. Eventually matters came to a head when her condition deteriorated but she refused to take the anti-psychotic medication, considered essential if she was to remain a patient in an adolescent psychiatric unit. She was seen by a consultant child psychiatrist who concluded that she was of sufficient maturity and understanding to comprehend the recommended treatment and was currently rational, but that should treatment (ie the medication) not be continued, her psychotic behaviour and suicidal tendencies were likely to return within days or weeks. Despite the opinion of her psychiatrist the court decided that she was not Gillick competent and thus could not give an informed refusal. No child who was 'only competent on a good day' could pass the Gillick test. As a result the court could authorize medication.

Ultimately the decision about a child's ability will rest on the health professional involved in the child's care. Note however, that some guidance is given in the current NHS Guidelines on consent (Chapter 2, para. 10). It recommends that a full note should be kept of the factors taken into account in assessing the child's capacity. Furthermore, where a child is seen alone, efforts should be made to persuade the child that his or her parents should be informed except when this is not in the child's interests.

It should also be noted that a court, but not a person with parental responsibility, can override a Gillick competent child's consent, the effect of which would be to prevent the proposed treatment being carried out.

Refusing consent

Just as with competent 16- and 17-year-olds, the right of Gillick competent children under 16 to withhold consent and refuse medical care (ie examination, assessment and treatment) can be overridden both by a court and a person with parental responsibility. In such cases it should be noted that the child's views are of the greatest importance, both legally and clinically, and their importance increases with the age and maturity of the child (see Re W above).

Not 'Gillick competent'

Children under 16 who do not have the capacity to make their own medical decisions may have consent given for them by anyone with parental responsibility, or the court. Once this has been obtained, treatment can be lawfully carried out providing it is in the child's best interests. In addition, for some potentially controversial procedures in the so-called 'special category', a court's permission may be necessary (see below).

Consent is not required in the following situations:

- emergencies – treatment can be carried out without consent if the treatment is necessary to safeguard the life and health of the child (providing the treatment does not go beyond the exigencies of the situation)

- exceptional circumstances – where the child has been abandoned or neglected by those with parental responsibility there is some authority for saying that consent is unnecessary (in such cases however the local authority is likely to take compulsory action and thereby acquire parental responsibility).

More problematic, however, are those cases, albeit rare, where a parent refuses to consent to treatment and there is no-one else with parental responsibility who is prepared to give the necessary consent. This happened in the case of Re E (Wardship: medical treatment) (1993) 1 FLR 179 when a 15-year-old Jehovah's Witness dying of leukaemia refused blood products. With treatment there was an 80 to 90% chance of full remission. An alternative treatment gave only a 60% chance of remission. Because of his refusal, which was supported by the boy's parents, the hospital adopted the alternative course of treatment and within two weeks his condition had deteriorated to the extent that his life was threatened. The hospital applied to court to treat the child as they considered necessary, including the transfusion of blood.

The court overrode both the parents' and the boy's refusal and gave the hospital permission to treat the boy as they considered necessary. In particular it was held that the boy was not Gillick competent, primarily because he had no realization of the full implications which lay before him in the process of dying, nor sufficient understanding and intelligence to comprehend the pain and distress he would suffer by refusing the treatment involving blood transfusions.

Note that NHS Guidelines (Chapter 2, para. 12) give clear advice on appropriate action when consent to urgent or life-saving treatment is refused. Where time permits, the court's permission should be obtained, otherwise it recommends that hospital authorities should rely on the clinical judgement of the relevant health professional after full discussion with the parents. In addition, written supporting evidence should be obtained from a colleague to the effect that the child's life is in danger if the treatment is withheld. The need to treat should also be discussed with parents in the presence of a witness who should counter-sign the record of the discussion in the clinical notes.

Role of the court

Health-related issues concerning children are most likely to be taken to court in the following types of situations:

- when disputes arise between parents and competent children concerning proposed medical treatment
- when parents and health professionals disagree on treatment for an incompetent child patient
- when a local authority disagrees with the proposed treatment for an incompetent child patient
- when the medical treatment sought has such serious implications (ie 'special category' cases) that it is appropriate to seek assistance from the courts

- when there is doubt about the validity of a minor's consent, or refusal of consent.

The cases which have commonly been taken to court in the past have involved abortion, contraception, sterilization and life-saving treatment (*see* below). However it should be noted that it is possible for any health-related issue to be taken to court, especially since there are now a number of different ways of initiating court proceedings, ie wardship, the court's inherent jurisdiction and the new Section 8 orders, notably the specific issue order and the prohibited steps order (*see* Chapter 4).

The court's powers

The court's decision is based on what it considers to be the child's best interests. Hence it may:

- override parental opposition to treatment and give permission for it to be carried out
- override a competent minor's refusal of consent (whether he or she is over or under 16)
- override any consent that has been given, whether by a parent or competent minor and thus prevent treatment being carried out
- authorize the withholding of life-saving procedures.

Extensive though these powers seem, they do have limits. In Re J (a minor) (medical treatment) (1992) 2 FLR 165, for example, it was decided that no court could require a health professional or health authority to adopt a course of treatment which was, in the bona fide clinical judgement of those concerned, contraindicated as not being in the best interests of the patient. Moreover, it is also clear that consent by itself creates no obligation to treat. This acts as a flak-jacket, protecting health professionals from civil or criminal liability, and means no health professional can be compelled to treat a child just because someone – whether the parents, the child or the court – has consented.

Consent and the Children Act 1989

So far the discussion has focused on the common law of consent. But what does the Children Act say about a child's consent to medical and psychiatric examinations and assessments? Many of the Act's provisions, notably those dealing with child protection, enable the court to include in court orders directions about medical and psychiatric examinations or other assessments.
    The orders in question are:

- interim care order
- interim supervision order
- full supervision order (this is the only order which can include directions about treatment)

- child assessment order
- emergency protection order.

But in all these instances the Act specifically states that children with 'sufficient understanding to make an informed decision' can refuse to submit to them. Does this mean that 'mature' minors have an absolute and conclusive right of veto in relation to these orders? Such an interpretation is clearly intended as far as the guidance documentation is concerned (*see* Guidance Vol. 1, para. 3.50–51). Furthermore, most commentators consider the courts would be unlikely to take away children's statutory right of informed refusal, especially since the Act only has a very specific and limited remit (ie with the exception of full supervision orders it appears only to apply to medical and psychiatric examination and assessment).

Finally, it should be noted that the Act gives no guidance on how a child's capacity is to be determined. It seems likely, therefore, that the principles used in ascertaining Gillick competence (*see* above) will apply. Ultimately, however, it is the health professionals involved in each case who must ascertain competence. As the guidance warns:

> 'directions by a court will not absolve a doctor or other person conducting the examination or assessment from his responsibility to satisfy himself that the child of sufficient age and understanding consents. He should not proceed if such consent is withheld but should arrange for the facts of the matter to be reported to the court which gave the directions as soon as possible, usually via the guardian at litem'. (Vol. 1, para. 3.51)

In cases where a child makes an informed refusal but no health-related directions have been given by the court it is advisable for reference to be made back to the court for guidance.

Abortion

The Abortion Act 1967 (as amended by the Human Fertilization and Embryology Act 1990) makes no special reference to girls who are minors but provides that abortion can be carried out provided certain conditions are complied with (*see* Appendix B). This means that a girl under 16 can give a valid consent to an abortion providing she:

- is 'Gillick competent' (ie understands the nature and consequences of what is involved, especially the risks attendant on abortion)
- cannot be persuaded either to inform her parents or allow them to be informed
- the abortion is lawful and in her best interests.

Competent young people of 16 and 17 have the same rights as adults to consent to medical treatment, including abortion (*see* Section 8 Family Law Reform Act 1969, above). When a girl under 18 is not competent consent must normally be given by a person with parental responsibility or the court, unless the operation is urgently needed to save the girl's life.

Less clear is the position of a competent girl under 18 refusing to have an abortion which parents or others, for example a local authority or health professional, consider necessary. So far, there have been no cases directly on this point although theoretically following Re W (see above) it seems that an abortion could be carried out in reliance on the consent of parents (or the court) despite the refusal of consent from the girl concerned. Whether a court would authorize an abortion in these circumstances is doubtful. One should also query whether even with the court's permission, a health professional would be willing to carry out an abortion on an unwilling and competent young person.

There have, however, been two important cases where girls wanted an abortion against their parents' wishes. The case of Re P (a minor) (1982) LGR 301 concerned a 15-year-old girl in care who lived in a mother and child unit with her 11-month-old son. She became pregnant for the second time and wanted an abortion (a decision supported by the local authority) to which her parents were vehemently opposed on religious grounds. Although there were a number of factors influencing the judge's decision to permit the abortion, the wishes of the girl herself were particularly persuasive. Moreover, given the local authority's inability to monitor the girl's sexual activities, the court also authorized that suitable internal contraceptive devices be fitted.

In the case Re B (Wardship) (abortion) (1991) 2 FLR 426 the girl at the centre of the dispute was 12. She became pregnant and wanted an abortion. Her decision was supported by the 16-year-old father and her grandparents who had brought her up but her mother opposed the termination. Medical evidence was conflicting but again the court overrode the mother's wishes and gave permission for the abortion to go ahead, not just because the girl wanted it but because the court thought it was in her best interests.

Contraception

Although the precise scope of the Gillick case remains uncertain, especially as regards the refusal of consent, contraceptive advice and treatment can be given to under-age girls, providing the guidelines laid down in the case are met. These guidelines, which have been incorporated in LAC 86(3) (Family Planning Services For Young People), state that contraceptive advice and treatment can be provided to young people under 16 without parental knowledge or consent, provided a doctor or other health professional is satisfied that:

- they understand the advice and have sufficient maturity to understand what is involved in terms of the moral, social and emotional implications
- they cannot be persuaded to inform their parents or allow them to be informed that advice is being sought
- they would be very likely to begin or to continue having sexual intercourse with or without contraceptive treatment
- without contraceptive advice or treatment their physical or mental health or both are likely to suffer

- their best interests require contraceptive advice, treatment or both without parental consent.

Competent 16- and 17-year-olds can give valid consent to contraceptive advice and treatment by virtue of Section 8 of the Family Law Reform Act 1969 (*see* above). Consent to contraceptive treatment on behalf of incompetent young people under 18 can be given by any person with parental responsibility and likewise by the court.

Sterilization

Certain forms of treatment within the so-called 'special category' raise such fundamental issues of law, ethics and medical practice that the court's prior permission is normally required. This includes sterilization to prevent pregnancy (and *inter vivos* organ donation for transplant) in respect of a minor.

The reasons for the court's involvement in sterilization cases are as follows:

- even though the operation can only be performed if it is in the minor's 'best interests' there may be greater risk of it being decided wrongly, such as for improper reasons or motives
- it should protect those who perform the operation from any subsequent legal liability
- it provides the best forum for bringing together and considering all the expert and other relevant evidence such as the minor's history, circumstances and foreseeable future, the risks and consequences of pregnancy, the risks and consequences of sterilization, the practicability of alternative precautions against pregnancy and any other relevant information.

The case of Re B (a minor) (sterilization) (1988) AC 199 is a good illustration of how the courts reach a decision. It concerned an epileptic girl of 17 who did not need protection under the Mental Health Act 1983 but was of low intelligence with a mental age of five or six. Sterilization was proposed for a variety of reasons: she was sexually mature but could not be placed on any effective contraceptive regime; she was said to be incapable of understanding (or learning) the causal connection between intercourse, pregnancy and childbirth; irregular menstruation meant that it would be difficult to detect or diagnose a pregnancy in time to terminate it easily; she would be likely to panic if pregnant and could not cope with labour; a caesarian section would not be appropriate since she had a high pain threshold and would probably pick at a wound and tear it open. Given all these factors it was decided that sterilization was in her best interests and could lawfully be performed.

While Re B is the most well known case concerning sterilization of minors, other less well publicized cases have also dealt with sterilization. In Re E (medical treatment) (1991) 2 FLR 585, for example, a hysterectomy was performed on a 17-year-old mentally retarded girl who suffered severe menstrual problems. The court held that its consent was not required for an operation – the inevitable and incidental effect of which is sterilization – provided it was carried out for therapeutic reasons (ie to treat a medical condition).

Treatment for handicapped infants

Until comparatively recently there have been few legal guidelines on appropriate treatment for handicapped newborn infants. But in the last decade three important cases have come before the courts which provide some guidance on how future cases would be decided.

Re B (a minor) (1981) 1 WLR 1421

This case concerned a baby girl born with Down's syndrome and an intestinal blockage which would be fatal within a few days unless urgent life-saving surgery was performed. If she had a successful operation her life expectancy could be about 20 to 30 years but B's parents refused to consent to surgery genuinely believing it was in her best interests to be allowed to die. The local authority made the child a ward of court.

The basic issue before the court was 'whether the life of the child was going to be so awful that in effect the child must be condemned to die, or whether her life was so imponderable that it would be wrong for her to be so condemned'. Unfortunately, one of the difficulties of the case was that there was no prognosis as to B's future – no-one could say whether she would suffer, nor to what extent her mental and physical defects would be apparent. Nonetheless, it was accepted that she would be very mentally and physically handicapped and would not have anything like a 'normal existence'.

The court authorized surgery and thus overruled the parents' wishes. Parental wishes were said to be never conclusive even though great weight should be attached to them. Essentially the reason for the decision was that the evidence before the court only established that if the operation took place and was successful, the child might live the normal life span of a Down's syndrome child with the handicaps and defects of such a child. Accordingly the court was not prepared to say that a 'life of that description should be extinguished'. In other words medical treatment could significantly improve the child's life, at least in the sense of extending her life expectancy.

Re C (a minor) (1989) 2 All ER 782

In this case the baby was born prematurely suffering from a serious form of hydrocephalus. At 16 weeks she was terminally ill and had massive physical and mental handicaps with blindness, probable deafness and spastic cerebral palsy of all four limbs. Her ultimate prognosis was one of hopelessness as she was dying and the only question was how soon this would happen. The central issue before the court was what treatment should be given if, as sooner or later was inevitable,

C suffered some infection or illness over and above the handicaps from which she was already suffering. For example, if it became impossible to feed her through a syringe should she be fed through a naso-gastric tube or intravenously? And should antibiotics be given if she developed an infection?

The court directed that C should receive treatment which was appropriate to her condition, ie to relieve her suffering rather than to achieve a short prolongation of her life. In effect this meant that it would not be necessary to prescribe antibiotics or to set up artificial feeding regimes simply to prolong her life.

The above two cases clearly represent different situations. When a baby is terminally ill the court will not order medical procedures to prolong life but when it is severely handicapped (although not intolerably so) and treatment can enable life to continue for an appreciable period subject to the severe handicap, then appropriate treatment should be given.

But how should the court resolve cases which can be said to lie between these two extremes, those where there might be a variety of handicaps, some treatable but others, perhaps the most painful, untreatable? The following case falls well within this middle category.

Re J (a minor) (1990) 3 All ER 930

Baby J was 13 weeks premature (weighing 1.1 kg at birth). By the time the case came to court he was five months old but had suffered recurrent convulsions and had been ventilated twice for long periods. He was now able to breathe independently but the long-term prognosis was very poor: he was likely to develop serious spastic quadraplegia, would be blind and deaf but would experience the same pain as a normal baby. His life expectancy was uncertain but he was expected to die before late adolescence.

The central question before the court was if he suffered further collapse should he be resuscitated again. Medical opinion was unanimous that in his present condition he should not be put back onto a mechanical ventilator. The court agreed, stating that J should be treated with antibiotics if he developed a chest infection but should not be reventilated if his breathing stopped unless those caring for him deemed it appropriate given the prevailing clinical situation.

Some general guidelines were also given in this case. Firstly, in deciding whether to direct that treatment (without which death would ensue from natural causes) need not be given to prolong life, the court had to perform a balancing exercise. This involved judging the quality of life the child would have to endure if given treatment and then deciding whether in all the circumstances such a life 'would be so afflicted as to be intolerable to that child'. Secondly, there was a strong presumption in favour of a course of action which would prolong life. Thirdly, the best interests test must be looked at from the child's point of view.

Medical records

Two recent statutes have given patients a legal right of access to health records kept both in computerized form and in manual form.

Access to Health Record Act 1990

This Act which came into force on 1 November 1991 applies to records kept in manual form. A health record is defined as any record which consists of information relating to the physical or mental health of an individual who can be identified from that information which has been made by or on behalf of a health professional in connection with the individual's care. This includes not only contents of the medical record envelope but also practice diaries and visit books. The term health professional is broadly defined and includes doctors, dentists, opticians, nurses, midwives, health visitors and various other paramedics.

The Act gives a right of application for access to the patient to whom the record relates and, in certain circumstances, other individuals. The Act also provides for the correction of inaccurate records. Access must be made in writing by, amongst others, the patient, someone appointed on the patient's behalf and in the case of a child under 16 any person with parental responsibility. If the applicant is a person with parental responsibility, access should not be given unless the health professional is satisfied that the child agrees, or is incapable of agreeing and access is in the child's best interests.

Patients under 16 can apply in their own right but access will only be given if the record holder is satisfied that they are capable of understanding the nature of the application.

Note that the Act does not guarantee access, as it can be wholly or partly refused on various grounds (ie disclosure would cause serious harm to the physical or mental health of the patient).

The Data Protection Act 1984

This Act applies to records held on computer. It is designed to ensure that relevant information is obtained fairly, kept up-to-date, securely stored and not disclosed to unauthorized persons. Individuals whose data is stored have a right to be supplied with a copy of the information relating to them. Requests for information must be made in writing. When a child applies it must be determined whether the child understands the nature of the request, if not then anyone with parental responsibility can make a request. Access is not unlimited and can be excluded in certain specified circumstances such as if the data is likely to cause serious harm.

Case studies

Case study 4

Delia is 13 and an only child. She lives with her elderly parents, Elsa and Fred, who are both in poor health. Elsa is crippled by arthritis and Fred has had several heart attacks. Delia has very few friends since she spends most of her time studying, caring for her parents and looking after the house. Recently, however, she has become friendly with Edward, a 16-year-old neighbour. Their relationship flourishes and soon Delia discovers she is pregnant. She hides the pregnancy from her parents for as long as possible though, as she is petrified of what they will say.

Although Delia and Edward want to get married and have children one day they both think they are much too young to have a child now, especially as they both hope to go to university. Therefore, they reluctantly decide that the pregnancy should be terminated. But when Elsa and Fred find out about their daughter's plans they go and see their GP and tell her that they will not consent to the abortion and will do everything possible to prevent it. They claim they are quite capable of caring for their grandchild and would not expect much, if any, help from Delia. The GP thinks that it is extremely unlikely that either Elsa or Fred could cope on their own if Delia left home, and certainly could not look after a young baby. But she is not certain about their rights, as parents, to prevent Delia terminating her pregnancy.

1. Does Delia have the right to give consent to an abortion?
2. Even if Delia can give a valid consent can her consent be overridden (ie can the abortion still be prevented) by Elsa and Fred, or anyone else?
3. Would it make any difference if Delia was 17?
4. What action could Fred or Elsa take to prevent the abortion?

Solutions

1. Even though Delia is only 13 she can give a valid consent to an abortion provided she is 'Gillick competent' (ie of sufficient age and understanding to comprehend the nature of an abortion and its implications). However, her pregnancy can only be terminated if she satisfies the criteria in the Abortion Act 1967.
2. If Delia is 'Gillick competent' her consent cannot be overridden by anyone with parental responsibility (ie Elsa or Fred). However, it could be overridden, and the abortion could be prevented, by a court if it considered an abortion contrary to Delia's best interests.
3. If Delia was 17 her right to consent to an abortion would be governed by Section 8 of the Family Law Reform Act 1969 which gives competent 16- and 17-year-olds the right to give valid legal consent to medical treatment. As with 'Gillick competent' under-16-year-olds however, such consent could be overridden by a court but not by Fred or Elsa.
4. Fred or Elsa would be advised to take a prohibited steps order to prevent the abortion.

Case study 5

Eli is a very active 15-year-old who loves all kinds of sports and is captain of his school football team. Recently he has been told that he is so good that with a little extra coaching he could possibly become a professional footballer. But whilst playing in a match one Saturday he suddenly falls over for no apparent reason and is rushed to hospital. After various preliminary X-rays and tests the hospital casualty officer suspects that Eli may have cancer.

When this diagnosis is confirmed and Eli is told, his main anxiety is about treatment. He is absolutely adamant that he will not have his leg amputated even though this is the recommended treatment for him and the one most likely to prolong his life. Without an active sports life Eli is convinced that life 'would not be worth living'. Eli's mother, Fran, thinks that his wishes should be respected but his father, Gary, disagrees. He thinks that his son is far too young to make such a major decision and that he should be able to consent to the amputation on his son's behalf.

1. Can hospital staff rely on Gary's consent to the amputation even though Eli and Fran both oppose it?
2. Would it make any difference if Eli was nearly 18?
3. What action could Eli himself take to resolve the issue?

Solutions

1. Even though a 'Gillick competent' young person under 16 can give valid consent it now seems that this capacity does not necessarily extend to refusing consent (at least not in relation to life-saving treatment). This means that anyone with parental responsibility, such as Gary, could authorize surgery. A court could also give consent. In non-urgent cases, though, surgery should be postponed until the dispute had been resolved, by court proceedings if necessary.
2. If Eli was nearly 18 then Section 8 of the Family Law Reform Act 1969 would apply. Although this does give competent 16- and 17-year-olds the statutory right to give valid consent, their right to refuse consent can be overridden by any person with parental responsibility, such as Gary, or a court. In other words, even if Eli was nearly 18 he may find his informed refusal overridden.
3. Eli could apply for a specific issue order. He does not have an automatic right to make the application but would first have to get the court's permission. Permission would only be given if the court was satisfied he had sufficient understanding to make the proposed application.

4

Court Orders in Family Proceedings

This chapter will consider the courts' powers under Part II of the Act to resolve disputes which are most likely to arise in 'private' family proceedings such as divorce and separation. A completely new set of orders has been created which are designed to prevent children becoming 'pawns in their parents' battles' – a not uncommon feature of previous legislation. Overall, the new scheme establishes a framework which, in theory, should encourage joint parenting and negotiated settlements by focusing on 'practical realities' rather than the legal status of parents or allocation of theoretical rights.

To ensure that the best arrangements can be made, the court is given a much more protective and inquisitorial role enabling it to control and manage cases more effectively. In addition a much wider group of people can now apply for any of the orders.

The scope and effect of the four Section 8 orders: residence, contact, prohibited steps and specific issue will be considered in turn. Note that all the orders can be varied or discharged by the court and they are automatically discharged by a care order. There are also extensive rights of appeal.

Residence orders

A residence order means an order 'settling the arrangements to be made as to the person with whom a child shall live'. Basically, the order names the person who is to look after the child, although it can also state where he should live as well. Residence orders are broadly similar to the old and no longer available care, control and custody orders but are far more flexible. Consequently they can be easily adapted to suit a wider range of living arrangements than was previously possible. This means that they will not only be used in the most usual arrangement – whereby a child lives most of the time with one parent – but can also encompass joint, shared care arrangements where the child's home is divided, not necessarily equally, between both parents and possibly other relatives.

The relationship between residence orders and parental responsibility

Existing parental responsibility is unaffected by the making of a residence order. Divorced parents thus retain it regardless of where or with whom their child lives.

Similarly an order will not affect an unmarried father's parental responsibility – acquired by virtue of a parental responsibility order of agreement – although the court can remove it from him.

However, to make sure that other people with residence orders, for example a grandmother, can have legal authority to make decisions about a child's up-bringing, the Act provides that whilst they are in force residence orders auto-matically confer parental responsibility. Note, however, that when the court makes an order in favour of an unmarried father it must also make a separate parental responsibility order. Furthermore, he will retain that responsibility until it is removed by the court, even if the residence order ceases.

The effect of these complex provisions is that in some cases parental respons-ibility could be shared between various different people at the same time. For example, a grandmother or foster parents and the child's parents. Furthermore all of them can exercise their parental responsibility independently, without any obligation to consult each other. No-one, however, can do anything that con-travenes a court order or statutory requirement.

In practice, of course, it is the person with actual day-to-day care of the child who has the greatest control. Moreover there are some aspects of parental responsibility which can never be acquired by non-parents. They cannot, for example, consent to a child's adoption, nor an order freeing the child for adoption, nor appoint a guardian. As long as a residence order is in force there are also restrictions on changing the child's surname and taking him or her out of the United Kingdom (see Section 13).

PRACTICE NOTES

Health professionals may be asked to advise on the suitability of proposed living arrangements and/or an applicant for a residence order.

Contact orders

A contact order 'requires the person with whom a child lives, or is to live, to allow the child to visit or stay with the person named in the order, or for that person and the child to have contact with each other'. In other words it compels the child's carer to permit visits or whatever type of contact is specified to the per-son(s) named in the order.

Contact orders replace access orders but are intended to be more child-centred, focusing on the child's right of contact rather than anyone else's. They are likely to be made when a child spends much more time with one parent than the other. However, 'contact' is expected to be very broadly interpreted. It is not confined to face-to-face experiences but can also include communication by letter, tele-phone and video tape etc.

If reasonable contact arrangements cannot be agreed by the parties themselves the court has wide powers to specify when, where and how they should take place. Contact between a child and his or her parent will rarely be refused, although this may be necessary in abuse cases. It is also worth noting that although the vast majority of disputes about contact involve parents other people, notably relatives, may also wish to obtain an order.

Section 8 contact orders can be used to regulate contact with children who are voluntarily provided with local authority accommodation but not in respect of children subject to a care order (the new care contact order under Section 34 applies instead, *see* Chapter 7).

PRACTICE NOTES

Health professionals may be asked to advise on the suitability of proposed contact arrangements and/or an applicant for an order.

Specific issue orders

This is a new order which did not exist in previous legislation. It means 'an order giving directions for the purpose of determining a specific question which has arisen, or which may arise, in connection with any aspect of parental responsibility for a child'. It is intended to replace wardship and enables the court to settle a single issue which has arisen (or is likely to arise), usually a major aspect of upbringing such as schooling, medical treatment, change of surname or religious education. Essentially, the order deprives parents of their legal right to make a particular decision and empowers the court to make it instead. Alternatively the court could decide that the issue should be determined by others. For example, in a case involving medical treatment the court could specify that the child should be treated by a named health professional.

Specific issue orders, which are expected to be used sparingly, can be made on their own or together with residence or contact orders but not 'with a view to achieving a result which could be achieved by making a contact or residence order'. In other words they must not be made as a back-door way of regulating where a child lives or whom he or she sees. Moreover they can only relate to actions which are within a parent's power.

PRACTICE NOTES

Specific issue orders are well suited to resolving contentious 'health care issues' which in the past would have been dealt with by wardship proceedings, as when parents of a young child are refusing consent to medical treatment or an HIV test for a symptomatic child.

Health professionals can themselves apply for an order. In extreme cases this may be the only way to protect a child. In some cases they may be required to give evidence.

Prohibited steps orders

This order directs that

> 'no step which could be taken by a parent in meeting his or her responsibility for a child, and which is of a kind specified in the order, shall be taken by any person without the consent of the court'.

It is therefore a 'negative' type of order which prevents something being done without permission. A prohibited steps order will usually be sought when one parent objects to something the other is doing. Like the specific issue order it did not exist in previous legislation and is concerned with a single aspect of upbringing. Examples of the kind of steps which could be 'prohibited' include taking a child out of the United Kingdom, contact with a particular person, medical treatment, change of surname or school and participation in a hazardous sport.

Despite the wide range of potential prohibitions, the order is not expected to be sought often and can only relate to action within a parent's power. It cannot be used to prevent one parent from contacting another. Nor can it be used as a substitute for a residence or contact order although it can be made in conjunction with them.

PRACTICE NOTES

Disputed 'health care steps' may well be the subject of a prohibited steps order in which case health professionals may be required to give evidence. It could be used, for example, to prevent cosmetic surgery, sterilization of a mentally handicapped child or male circumcision.

Health professionals can themselves apply for an order as possibly the only way a child can be protected in extreme cases.

Additional powers

To ensure maximum flexibility the courts have wide powers to specify in considerable detail the precise terms of any order. They can give directions or impose conditions, for example as to the frequency, location or duration of a contact order. These additional powers could be especially useful where a child is cared for by someone who is opposed to a certain form of medical treatment since a condition could be included in a residence order, for example that the carer will inform someone who will consent to treatment should the need arise.

Duration of orders

Normally all the orders will end when the child is 16, although they may be discharged or cease automatically before then. In exceptional circumstances, such as where a child is mentally or physically handicapped, they may be extended until the child is 18.

When will a Section 8 order be granted?

In deciding whether or not to make an order, or to vary or discharge one, the court must apply the principles set out in Section 1. These are that the child's welfare is the paramount consideration, the welfare check list, the non-intervention principle and the presumption against delay.

It is also important to note that a court can make any of the orders in proceedings brought specifically for that purpose (sometimes called 'freestanding' proceedings) or as part of other family proceedings such as divorce or 'domestic violence' and injunction cases, adoption and care proceedings.

The position of local authorities

Although it is likely that Section 8 orders will primarily be used to resolve private family disputes there may be occasion, especially in health-related disputes, when local authorities will wish to use them. For example, to prevent proposed medical treatment, to obtain the court's permission for controversial treatment or to ensure that a parent allows a child to be examined. Consequently the Act allows them to apply (with the court's permission) for either a specific or prohibited step order, providing they are not sought as an indirect 'back-door' way of either obtaining the care, supervision or accommodation of a child, or of gaining parental responsibility. In no circumstances, though, can local authorities apply for a residence or contact order (nor can either of these be made in their favour).

There are also restrictions on the use of Section 8 orders when a child is in care. Only a residence order can be made, the effect of which is to discharge the care order (a care order also discharges any existing Section 8 order). The intention here is to prevent parents using the Section 8 'menu' as a way of challenging how a local authority exercises its powers.

Who can apply for an order?

The Act has considerably widened access to the courts so as to give anyone who is genuinely interested in the child's welfare the opportunity to initiate proceedings. But to protect families from unwarranted interference and inappropriate applications various 'hurdles' are imposed. The broad effect of these fairly complex provisions is to permit the court itself to make orders on its own initiative and to divide other applicants into three groups.

Group 1: those entitled to apply for any Section 8 order

This group has automatic rights to apply for any order. It includes parents whether married or not, guardians and any person who has a residence order. Certain other people are also entitled to apply as of right to vary or discharge any order, *see* Section 10(6).

Group 2: those entitled to apply for residence and contact orders

This group is only entitled to apply as of right for residence or contact orders. It includes people who have such close links with the child that it is unlikely that unmeritorious applications would be made, most likely anyone to whom the child has been a 'child of the family' such as step-parents; anyone who has looked after the child for at least three years or more; anyone who has the consent of certain people namely, all those with a residence order or parental responsibility; or the local authority if the child is in care under a care order.

Group 3: those who require the court's leave

This category is potentially very wide as it allows anyone, such as grandparents, relatives or 'strangers', to apply for any Section 8 order. But they must first get the court's permission. In deciding whether to give leave the court must consider several matters, including the applicant's connection with the child, any risk of disruption to the child's life and where the child is being looked after by the local authority, its plans for the child's future, and the wishes and feelings of the parents.

Note that children themselves can also apply for any order, providing they have 'sufficient understanding' to make the application. Although local authority foster parents can also apply for orders they are subject to various conditions which do not apply to other applicants.

Other 'private' court orders

Although this chapter has focused on Section 8 orders, the Act also deals with other private law orders. These are:

- family assistance orders: new style orders which enable short-term support (ie mediation services) to be provided when families need help to overcome problems associated with divorce or separation
- financial orders: Section 15 and Schedule 1 contain various provisions – none of which are new – governing financial support for children
- guardians: substantial reforms are made to guardianship law, notably the appointment of guardians and the legal effects of guardianship.

Wardship

Private disputes about residence, contact or other aspects of upbringing are now expected to be resolved by the Section 8 'menu' rather than the wardship jurisdiction. Nevertheless, wardship operates alongside the new scheme and can be used as an alternative procedure, except by local authorities. In practice – partly because wardship is expensive – its use is likely to be restricted to very complex or unusual cases.

Case studies

Case study 6

Fay is 11 years old and lives with her mother, Gloria. Last year Fay's parents were divorced and a residence order was granted to Gloria. Fay's father, Hiram, regularly sees her, however, as she stays with him every alternate weekend except when he is away working. One of the main reasons for the divorce was the fact that Gloria became a Jehovah's Witness and although Hiram is happy for Fay to live with Gloria he is very anxious about what would happen if Fay ever needed a blood transfusion and he was not able to give consent, for example, because he was away working and did not know Fay needed one. On the many occasions they have discussed this Gloria has made it quite clear that she would never authorize a blood transfusion for Fay, even if her life was in danger.

1. Is there any way that when the residence order is granted the court could ensure that consent to a transfusion could be obtained?
2. If the need for a transfusion arose and Hiram could not be contacted what should the hospital do?
3. If, when Fay is staying with Hiram, she is involved in an accident and needs surgery can Hiram authorize treatment?

4. If Fay's grandmother has a residence order and Fay needs medical treatment can her grandmother authorize it?

Solutions

1. The court has wide powers to attach conditions and directions to residence orders enabling it to settle current disputes and anticipate future ones. It can therefore make it a condition of the residence order that should the need for a blood transfusion arise Gloria must contact Hiram and inform him of the situation so that he can give the necessary consent. Alternatively it could settle the dispute by a specific issue order.

2. Hospital staff can transfuse Fay without obtaining any prior consent, providing it is an emergency and urgent treatment is necessary to save her life. In less urgent cases the issue should be resolved by a specific issue order (applied for, if necessary, by the health authority).

3. Even though Hiram does not have a residence order he still retains his parental responsibility. This means that he has an independent right to consent to medical treatment unless this has been curtailed in some way by the Children Act (eg by a specific issue order or prohibited steps order).

4. When a residence order is granted in favour of a person who is not a child's parent or guardian then that person has parental responsibility for as long as the residence order exists. This means that Fay's grandmother shares parental responsibility with Fay's parents and has an independent right to give consent to medical treatment. Note, however, that if such treatment is the subject of dispute and treatment is not urgently required it should be postponed until the dispute is resolved, by court proceedings if necessary.

Case study 7

Gavin is an eight-year-old Down's syndrome boy who also suffers from a congenital heart defect. Corrective surgery, involving only a 5 to 10% risk of mortality is proposed to avoid a painful, degenerative process, resulting in premature death in approximately 20 years, but Gavin's father, Harry, refuses his consent to surgery. Harry is nearing retirement age and is in very poor health himself. He has looked after Gavin himself since his wife died in a car accident four years previously but doubts whether he can care properly for Gavin for much longer.

Gavin's GP and the consultant paediatrician feel that Harry's wishes should be respected as he has looked after Gavin all his life and should know what is best for him. But Ingrid, another paediatrician feels that a court should intervene and decide what is the best treatment for Gavin.

1. Can Ingrid start court proceedings under the Children Act to resolve the dispute?
2. Which court order should she apply for?
3. Is she automatically entitled to start proceedings?
4. What principles will the court apply in deciding the case?

Solutions

1. Yes, she can apply for a Section 8 order.
2. The most appropriate order would be a specific issue order.
3. Ingrid does not have an automatic right to apply for an order but must obtain the court's leave. In deciding whether to grant permission for the application the court must consider the nature of the proposed application, Ingrid's connection with Gavin, and any risk there might be of the application disrupting his life to such an extent that he would be harmed by it.
4. As with all Section 8 orders the court's paramount consideration will be Gavin's welfare. The court must also consider the welfare check list, the non-intervention principle and presumption against delay.

Case study 8

Heidi is nearly 16 years old and the second of five children. She suffers from extreme expressive aphasia and is described as 'moderately' retarded. Heidi has some learning skills but to a limited level. Her mother, Iris, thinks that one day she might be able to carry out the mechanical duties of a mother, albeit under supervision, but would never be capable of being a mother in any other sense.

From Monday to Friday Heidi lives in local authority residential accommodation but she returns home every weekend. Home is a very small maisonette which is over-crowded and in need of substantial repair. Recently, Heidi has become very friendly with a young man, a situation which greatly troubles Iris as she fears that Heidi might become pregnant and, since she would never be able to cope with motherhood, the responsibility would fall on her. Since Iris, who is in poor health herself, was deserted by her husband five years ago she has to work very long hours and feels she could not possibly care for another young child.

This is why Iris decides that Heidi ought to be sterilized, a decision supported by both her GP and the consultant gynaecologist. Heidi is therefore booked into hospital for the operation to be carried out in two days' time. It is then that Jenny, the practice nurse, who has come to know Heidi very well over the last few years, decides that she must take urgent action to prevent her being sterilized, at least until a further opinion can be obtained.

1. What proceedings could Jenny start?
2. Does she need the court's permission to make her application?
3. If Heidi's father returned and wanted to look after her (against Iris' wishes) what order should he seek?

Solutions

1. Jenny could apply for a prohibited steps order under Section 8 of the Children Act.
2. As Jenny does not have an automatic right to start proceedings she will have to get the court's permission (for the relevant criteria *see* Case study 7 (3) above).

3. Heidi's father would have to seek a residence order which he has an automatic right to apply for because he is a parent.

Case study 9

Ian is eight years old. He was admitted to hospital last week following a serious car accident. It is likely that he will be there for another three weeks at least. His parents, who are not married, separated several months previously and a few days ago one of the nurses, Josette, noticed that Ian was very upset when his mother left after visiting him. He was again distressed after her visit the following day and when Josette asked Ian what was the matter he said that he desperately wanted to see his father, Kalef, but his mother was doing all she could to stop him from coming. Josette and other hospital staff think that Ian needs to see his father, especially as he is likely to spend a number of weeks in hospital.

1. What court order should Kalef apply for if he wants to see Ian?
2. What difference will it make if he does not have parental responsibility?
3. Will hospital staff be involved in the proceedings?

Solutions

1. Kalef should apply for a contact order under Section 8 of the Children Act which, as Ian's father, he can apply for as of right.
2. If Kalef does not have parental responsibility he still has an automatic right to apply for a contact order (likewise other Section 8 orders) because he is Ian's father. Therefore, it makes no difference whether he has parental responsibility or not.
3. In deciding whether to grant the contact order, Ian's welfare will be the court's paramount consideration. It will also consider the non-intervention principle, the welfare check list and the no-delay principle. Josette and other hospital staff who have had contact with Ian may be asked for their opinion as to whether contact with Kalef would benefit Ian and especially in ascertaining his wishes, feelings and emotional needs.

5

Local Authority Support for Children and Families

Part III of the Act covers the responsibilities of local authorities towards children and their families. It gives them a wide range of duties and powers aimed at supporting the family and ensuring that children can be brought up at home. Although many of these responsibilities existed in previous legislation others have been replaced, substantially amended or supplemented and some are completely new. Overall the reformed scheme has two broad objectives.

First, it aims to unify and rationalize the law. Previously local authorities had a number of overlapping obligations which derived from two very different sources: child care legislation and health and welfare legislation. As a result, service provision was patchy and unco-ordinated and there were wide regional variations both in policy and practice. By bringing together the two streams of law into one statute, local authorities should be able to provide a more integrated, efficient and coherent service.

The second aim is to encourage greater 'take-up' of services by emphasizing their positive benefits and advantages, and role in keeping families together. Under the old scheme some services, notably voluntary accommodation, had a very negative image and were regarded as stigmatizing, intrusive and threatening. They were also strongly associated with parental failure and inadequacy. By contrast, the new framework seeks to ensure that families needing help should receive a positive response which supports and supplements their efforts rather than marginalizes or undermines their role and authority. For the first time too, specific reference is made to the need to take account of children's religious, racial, cultural and linguistic backgrounds.

Underlying the new scheme is the pervasive theme of 'partnership', not just between local authorities, parents and children but also between local authority social service departments, other local authority departments such as health, housing and education, other agencies and the voluntary and private sector. Although the concept of partnership is not new, being based on well-established beliefs, the Act attempts to give it more statutory force, largely by strengthening the rights of parents and children to be consulted and informed and requiring a co-operative and collaborative approach to the provision of services.

Duties and powers

The responsibilities imposed upon local authorities, which include not only social services but also other departments such as health and education, are divided into two categories: duties and powers. Duties are compulsory. In other words there is a legal obligation to carry them out. They can be either absolute (an authority 'must' or 'shall' do something) or qualified (an authority 'shall take reasonable steps' as 'they consider appropriate' or 'as are reasonably practicable'). Unsurprisingly local authorities have very wide discretion in interpreting and exercising their qualified duties. Duties can also be either 'general' or 'specific'. General duties tend to be very open-ended and imprecise, whereas specific duties are considerably narrower and more detailed.

Powers are functions that local authorities can exercise if they so choose. In other words they are not legally obliged to carry them out. Powers are usually recognizable by the word 'may' and are very similar in effect to qualified duties.

Who is entitled to local authority services? Most duties and powers are targeted towards children in need (*see* below). But there are some which are owed (or can be given) to all children. This chapter will deal with each group separately. Similarly, day care services and the provision of accommodation will be dealt with separately from other services.

Children in need

According to Section 17 a child in need is one:

- who is unlikely to achieve or maintain, or to have the opportunity of achieving or maintaining, a reasonable standard of health or development without the provision of services by a local authority
- whose health or development is likely to be significantly impaired, or further impaired, without the provision of such services
- who is disabled.

The word 'disabled' is further defined to mean 'blind, deaf or dumb, suffering from a mental disorder, substantially and permanently handicapped by illness, or congenital deformity, or suffering some other disability as may be prescribed'.

'Development' means physical, intellectual, emotional, social or behavioural development and 'health' means physical or mental health. Points worth noting about this definition follow.

First, it is deliberately wide to reinforce the emphasis on preventive support and services to families, and has three distinct categories, namely reasonable standard of health and development, significant impairment of health or development, and disablement. Secondly, it includes children with disabilities for the first time in child care legislation. Thirdly, it includes children who are already suffering from a low standard of health or development as well as those who might be in that position in the future unless preventive action is taken.

General duty to children in need

Local authorities have a general duty to safeguard and promote the welfare of children within their area who are in need and so far as is consistent with that duty, promote their upbringing by their families, by providing a range and level of services appropriate to their needs.

Arguably this general duty is broader than in previous legislation, even though it is owed to a more restricted category of children. But in keeping with the Act's overall strategy their welfare is the primary objective. Nevertheless it is clear that local authorities are not expected to meet every individual need, nor to make up deficiencies in families' incomes or take over the role of the social security system. Rather their role is to 'identify the extent of need and then make decisions on the priorities for service provision in their area in the context of that information and their statutory duties' (Vol. 2, para. 2.11).

The following additional points should also be noted:

1. The services provided and the numbers they can serve are largely left to the local authority's discretion. Each authority can therefore decide its own level and scale of services and the ones which will be given priority.
2. Local authorities do not have to be the sole providers of services as the Act allows them both to facilitate provision by others (in particular, voluntary organizations) and to arrange for others to act on their behalf (eg day care provision).
3. Services may be provided not just to children but also to the family generally or to any individual member of it. 'Family' in this context is broadly defined and includes 'any person who has parental responsibility or with whom the child has been living'. It can therefore include non-relatives.
4. Local authorities can provide assistance in kind or in cash. This power was first introduced nearly 30 years ago but has been recast and supplemented. Assistance in kind can cover the provision of accommodation as well as clothing, furniture etc. Cash payments can only be paid in 'exceptional circumstances'.

Collaboration and co-operation

Despite local authorities having prime responsibility for co-ordinating and providing services to children in need, the Act requires a 'corporate approach' to the provision of services. Co-operation between authorities and other bodies is now given statutory force by Section 27 which allows local authorities to request the help of health, education and housing authorities in performing their functions under Part III. Once help is requested the other authority or body must comply 'if it is compatible with its own statutory or other duties and obligations and does not unduly prejudice the discharge of any of its functions'.

PRACTICE NOTES

District health authorities, NHS trusts and family health services authorities must collaborate and co-operate with local authorities (and other authorities and bodies) at all levels including strategic, middle-management and practitioner. This means that health professionals must:

- liaise with other agencies in identifying, assessing and meeting children's health needs and promoting their upbringing by their families
- establish new organizational links rather than relying on ad hoc arrangements.

In deciding how to co-operate, health professionals must be guided by their own clinical judgement and the extent to which any purchaser-provider system may affect their statutory obligations.

How is the general welfare duty to be met?

Section 17 gives local authorities a broad 'umbrella' duty. How they are to discharge it is, however, spelt out in considerable detail elsewhere in the Act, notably Part 1 of Schedule 2. This very important schedule lists the wide range of services which can, and in some cases must, be provided. Some are 'preventive' and aimed at keeping children out of court and preventing their admission to care, whilst others are 'supportive' and aimed at supporting children at home or encouraging family re-unification. There are 11 provisions in all, some of which apply to all children and not just those in need. In summary they are as follows.

Identification of children in need

The new duty compels local authorities to 'take reasonable steps to identify the extent to which there are children in need within their area'. Although it is a qualified duty it is very important since it is the 'trigger' or 'gateway' to a package of services, including day care and accommodation.

Official guidance stresses that the child's needs include physical, emotional and educational needs according to his or her age, sex, race, religion, culture and language and the capacity of the current carer to meet those needs (Vol. 2, para. 2.4).

PRACTICE NOTES

Health professionals will need to work with local (and other) authorities in:

- agreeing the criteria by which children are defined as 'in need', especially in relation to such concepts as 'reasonable standard' of health or development and 'significant' or 'further impairment'

- identifying those children who do not come within the definition of 'disabled' – because they are partially sighted, hard of hearing, temporarily handicapped or have conditions which do not lead to handicap while controlled by drugs etc – but who could come within the other definitions of 'need' if their condition impairs their health or development
- developing strategies and systems which both seek out children in need and encourage children and their families to come forward
- agreeing mechanisms through which information can be transferred between agencies
- making appropriate referrals, via agreed health authority protocols, to social services departments.

Publicity and the provision of information

A new absolute duty is imposed on local authorities to publicize the services they provide and, where appropriate, those provided by others. They must also take 'reasonable steps' to ensure that those who might benefit from the services receive appropriate information. This duty supplements duties under the Chronically Sick and Disabled Persons Act 1970 to inform persons with disabilities, on request, of relevant services provided by them or by voluntary organizations.

The duty is intended to increase interest in and awareness of relevant services and enable parents to make informed choices about available facilities. Publicity material is expected to be sensitively presented, jargon free, clear and accessible to all groups in the community. It should also take account of linguistic and cultural factors and the needs of people with communication difficulties.

PRACTICE NOTES

Health professionals can contribute by:

- providing advice on the preparation of publicity material, particularly where the information is directed at children with disabilities
- publishing those services in which they play a key role, as in child development/ district handicap teams and community mental handicap or learning disability teams as well as child health surveillance programmes and other support groups
- obtaining relevant information and disseminating it where appropriate.

Assessment of children's needs

Surprisingly the Act does not impose any obligation on local authorities to assess children in need, but the duty to identify such children implicitly requires them to develop clear assessment procedures. Instead it says that they may assess a child's needs at the same time as any other assessment is being carried out under the Chronically Sick and Disabled Persons Act 1970, the Education Act 1981, the Disabled Persons (Services, Consultation and Representation) Act 1986, or any other enactment.

This provision is intended to facilitate assessment and make it more effective and less traumatic. In the past it was not uncommon for children to be subjected to a confusing variety of procedures. Now the framework exists for assessments under the Act to be combined with those under other legislation. Detailed guidance is given about how assessments should be made (*see* Vol. 2, paras. 2.7–9).

In particular assessments should be undertaken in 'an open way' and involve not just the child and those caring for him but also any other 'significant persons'. Local authorities are also expected to take account of the particular needs of the child in relation to health, development, disability, education, religious persuasion, racial origin, cultural and linguistic background.

PRACTICE NOTES

Co-operation and collaboration are key features of the new emphasis on multi-disciplinary assessments – to which health professionals are expected to contribute. In particular by:

- ensuring that children are seen 'in the round' whether their particular needs are for educational, health or social care
- ensuring that a child's health needs are effectively assessed, ie in a non-stigmatizing way and pitched at the appropriate level
- assessing the extent to which a child's health needs (in addition to other needs such as disability and emotional and physical development) are being met by existing services to the family or child and which agencies' services are best suited to those needs
- contributing to the planning process which follows assessment by identifying and advising how the child's health and overall development needs can best be met.

Provision for children living with their families and maintenance of the family home

Local authorities are required to make a range of services available 'as they consider appropriate' to support children at home. The following services are specifically mentioned: advice, counselling and guidance; home help; occupational, social, cultural or recreational activities; assistance towards holidays and transport or assistance with travel expenses to facilitate use of services. In addition, when children are living apart from their families, local authorities must take steps to reunite them with their families or promote contact between them.

PRACTICE NOTES

Health professionals may have a crucial role in ensuring the effective support of 'vulnerable' children at home or facilitating their rehabilitation, for example advice and counselling on health-related issues or occupational therapy.

Services for children with disabilities

Although 'disabled' children come within the definition of children in need and can thus benefit from the range of services mentioned above, the Act makes extra provision for them by imposing two additional responsibilities on local authorities. These are:

- the duty to maintain a register for disabled children
- the duty to provide services designed to minimize their disabilities and give them the opportunity to lead lives which are as normal as possible.

For further details of these duties *see* Chapter 11.

Duties and powers to all children

The responsibilities of local authorities are principally directed towards children in need, but some preventive services apply to all children, whether in need or not. Local authorities are required to:

- take reasonable steps, through the provision of services, to prevent children within their area from suffering ill-treatment or neglect and to inform other authorities about children likely to suffer harm
- take reasonable steps to reduce the need for various proceedings (ie care, criminal or wardship proceedings)
- encourage children not to commit criminal proceedings
- avoid the need to use secure accommodation
- provide such family centres as they consider appropriate (*see* detailed guidance in Vol. 2, para. 3.18–24).

In addition, local authorities can help alleged abusers to obtain alternative accommodation in order to protect children suffering, or children likely to suffer ill-treatment.

PRACTICE NOTES

Health professionals have a key role to play:

- in identifying those children who are suffering or who are likely to suffer harm, ill-treatment or neglect and alerting local authorities to the need for support and assistance
- advising local authorities as to the provision of family centres and, where appropriate, providing relevant services.

Day care

The need for good quality day care services has long been recognized, but in the past provision was largely left to the discretion of individual authorities. Consequently, regional variations both in the standard and availability of services were considerable. The Act establishes a new statutory framework which is designed to improve the provision of day care services and ensure that they are regularly monitored and reviewed. Local authorities are given a range of responsibilities which include a new duty to provide day care for children in need, comprehensive review obligations and new regulatory powers and duties.

Day care is broadly defined in the Act to mean 'any form of care or supervised activity provided for children in the day whether or not provided on a regular basis'. It includes pre-school services and activities for school children.

Pre-school provision

Section 18 obliges local authorities to provide day care 'as is appropriate' for children in need who are under five and not yet attending school. This can include nurseries, play groups, parent/toddler groups, toy libraries, drop-in centres, play-buses, child-minding services and befriending services. Facilities can be provided either by the local authority itself or by other organizations but must have regard to the different racial groups to which the children belong.

Local authorities also have the power, but are not obliged, to provide day care services to children under five who are not in need.

Activities for school children

In addition, local authorities must provide 'appropriate' care or supervised activities for school-aged children in need outside school hours or during the school holidays. For example, out of school clubs, holiday schemes and special interest activities such as sports clubs.

These services can also be provided for school-aged children who are not in need, but again this is a power which local authorities do not have to exercise.

PRACTICE NOTES

Health professionals may be the first to identify the need for day care provision, for example, referral to a befriending service could provide effective preventive support. Similarly, services like the Portage scheme could benefit parents of children with disabilities.

Health professionals may also be asked to provide 'support services', such as advice, training, guidance and counselling, for people working in day care settings.

Review of day care

The Act imposes a new duty on local authorities to review every three years not only the day care they themselves provide but also child-minding facilities and other day care for the under-eights in their area. The review process must be conducted with the local education authority as a 'joint exercise' and its results must be published. Detailed guidance on how it should be carried out is contained in Volume 2 Chapter 9.

PRACTICE NOTES

Effective review involves multi-agency co-operation and collaboration. In particular, local authorities should consult with relevant health authorities and health boards, consider their representations, and take into account primary health care interests.

Health professionals should contribute to the review process by:

- identifying how existing services could be improved by providing information on their quality and availability and the extent to which they are reaching children in need
- ensuring that services are developed that recognize and reflect the interdependence of the education, care and health needs of children
- considering how primary health care can be improved, for example through developing health promotion activities, making arrangements for child health surveillance or providing advice and developmental checks in more effective and efficient ways
- ensuring that reports of the review are made available by putting relevant notices in clinics, health centres, doctors' surgeries and hospitals.

Accommodation

Children may need to live away from home for a variety of reasons but under the old law this service (now used by about 20 000 children each year) was very unpopular. There were three main problems. First, the legal position of children in 'voluntary care', as it was then called, was unclear, as were the rights and responsibilities of parents and local authorities. Secondly, the distinction between voluntary care and compulsory care was blurred. It was not uncommon, for example, for voluntary care to 'drift' into compulsion as a result of a very controversial administrative procedure (the infamous Section 3 resolution). Thirdly, the service had a very negative image and was invariably seen as a 'last resort' crisis solution.

The main priority therefore was to establish a framework which clarified and safeguarded parents' rights, enhanced their responsibility and authority and transformed voluntary accommodation into a positive, responsive and consumer led 'back-up' service which families could choose or reject 'without pressure or prejudice' and which would help maintain the child within the family in the long-term. Achieving these aims required radical reforms. These included a change of terminology, replacing 'voluntary care' with the term 'provision of accommodation'; abolishing the Section 3 resolution; strengthening parents' and children's rights to participate and be consulted in decision-making processes; ensuring that parents retained their responsibility; and finally emphasizing the co-operative 'partnership' nature of the arrangement.

The new strategy was primarily implemented in Section 20 which, unsurprisingly, distinguishes between children in need and other children. Local authorities must provide accommodation for children in need within their area if there is no-one with parental responsibility for them, if they are lost or have been abandoned or if their carers are unable to care for them whether or not permanently and for whatever reason. They must also provide accommodation for young people in need of 16 or 17 but only if their welfare is likely to be 'seriously prejudiced'. This provision generally applies to teenage run-aways.

Local authorities also have a discretion to provide accommodation for other children in their area if it would safeguard and promote their welfare. A similar power exists in respect of 16- to 21-year-olds who can be accommodated in community homes.

Legal consequences of the provision of accommodation

As the provision of accommodation is designed to reflect a 'respite' care philosophy and to provide a non-stigmatizing, support service for families under stress, fundamental changes have been made to its legal effects. These include the following:

1. *Parental responsibility.* The local authority does not acquire parental responsibility. This remains with whoever had it before the child was accommodated (usually the parents). However, the authority may do what is reasonable 'to safeguard and promote the child's welfare'. Note also that the Act prevents accommodation being provided where any person with parental responsibility who is willing and able to provide or arrange for the child's accommodation objects. This veto does not apply, however, when a child over 16 agrees to be

accommodated and when the holder of a residence order (or anyone who has care of the child in wardship) wants accommodation to be provided.

2. *Removal from accommodation.* Any person with parental responsibility can remove the child from accommodation at any time without giving the local authority any prior notice. (Under the old law 28 days notice had to be given in certain circumstances.) Again though, 16-year-olds can refuse to be removed and those with residence orders and wardship rights can also restrict removal. In cases where it is necessary to prevent a child's removal, various options are available to a local authority. It could, for example, apply for a care or emergency protection order. Other 'retaining' measures could also be invoked if necessary.

3. *Agreements.* A central element in the philosophy of partnership is the use of negotiated agreements. Local authorities are now obliged to enter into such agreements which contain detailed individualized plans, with the parents of each accommodated child. The contents of the agreement are prescribed in regulations (*see* Chapter 9).

4. *Consultation.* Before providing accommodation local authorities have a qualified duty to ascertain a child's wishes and give them due consideration, having regard to his or her age and understanding.

PRACTICE NOTES

The statutory requirement of inter-agency co-operation applies as much to the provision of accommodation as other local authority Part III functions. Health professionals should collaborate and liaise with the local authority and other relevant agencies in:

- identifying and assessing children's need for accommodation, especially when the accommodation requirements are related to a child's special needs or a parent's disability
- agreeing the criteria by which young people over 16 should qualify for accommodation.

Case studies

Case study 10

Jason is nearly three years old and his sister, Karen, is ten. They live with their mother, Leila, and her boyfriend, Martin. Although Leila tries very hard to care for her children she is finding it very difficult, partly because she has so little income but mainly because her home is very damp, as well as being in need of substantial repair. It is also very expensive to heat and so is often very cold. Martin has very little to do with the children as he is a long-distance lorry driver and rarely at home for any length of time. Leila is also having problems feeding Jason who is a very faddy eater. She worries too about disciplining Karen who has very few toys or games, no space to play in and no easy access to appropriate outside facilities.

When Norma, the health visitor, visits the children she is particularly concerned about Jason whose development seems well below average for his age. His failure to thrive is later confirmed following a detailed assessment. Karen, on the other hand, seems to be developing satisfactorily but Norma thinks she could benefit from some kind of local authority support, especially after school, when she just sits listlessly at home. Norma discusses her concerns with the GP who agrees that Jason, but not Karen, needs some kind of support services.

1. Are Jason and Karen entitled to local authority services?
2. If so, which ones?
3. Are Norma and the GP obliged to participate in the assessment process?
4. What if Norma thinks the services offered are inappropriate or inadequate?

Solutions

1. Local authorities must take reasonable steps to identify children who come within the definition of 'in need' within their area. So if Jason or Karen are considered 'unlikely to achieve or maintain, or to have the opportunity of achieving or maintaining, a reasonable standard of health or development without service provision; or their health or development is likely to be impaired, or further impaired without such services', then the local authority have a duty to safeguard and promote their welfare by providing a range of services.

   Whilst Jason is likely to be considered 'in need' Karen may not. Despite this certain services may still be provided (*see* 2 below).

2. Some form of day care support might be particularly useful for Jason – such as a place at a nursery or child-minding or playgroup facilities. Temporary accommodation or rehousing might also be useful if the family's housing problems are the main cause of Jason's failure to thrive. Other appropriate facilities might include advice, counselling and guidance at a family centre.

   If Karen was not considered a child 'in need' the local authority have the option of providing day care services for her (the most appropriate being some kind of out-of-school club or activity and a place on a holiday scheme).

3. Although the primary responsibility for identifying and assessing children 'in need' lies with the local authority (ie social services) other relevant authorities, notably health, housing and voluntary agencies are expected to contribute where appropriate so that a co-ordinated package of services can be planned and then provided.

   This means that both Norma and the GP should contribute to the assessment of Jason and Karen by providing relevant information about the family's situation and participating in a full assessment of the children, especially their health and developmental needs.

4. If Norma thinks the services provided are inadequate (or they are not provided at all) she should first discuss her concerns with the local authority. If her concerns are not taken seriously she could consider with Leila the possibility of a complaint being made under the representations and complaints procedures which all local

authorities are now obliged to set up. It may even be appropriate or necessary for Norma herself to make the complaint, providing she could persuade the local authority that she had 'sufficient interest' in the children's welfare.

Case study 11

Lorna is 14 years old and has been voluntarily provided with accommodation by the local authority for the last six months while her mother, Mona, tries to sort out her long-term drinking problem. She has not seen her father, Neil, for over two months as he is working hundreds of miles away. He keeps in contact with her though, telephoning her regularly and seeing her when he can.

Neil and Mona were divorced a year ago but no residence order was granted to either of them. Lorna is now happily settled with foster parents, Mr and Mrs Bhutta, and has recently told them she would like to carry on living with them even when her mother gets better.

Several days ago Lorna, who suffers from asthma, had a serious attack and was taken to hospital. Just as she is about to leave, Mona, who seems to be drunk, turns up and decides that Lorna should come with her immediately. Lorna is very distressed and pleads with hospital staff to let her go home with Mr and Mrs Bhutta or at least contact her father so that she can live with him. Lorna's GP thinks that it would be best for Lorna to stay with her foster parents.

1. Does Mona have the right to insist on Lorna's immediate return?
2. Could Neil insist that Lorna returns with him? Would he still have this right if he and Mona had never married?
3. Does Lorna have the right to have her wishes taken into account?
4. Does Lorna's GP have any right to be consulted about where she should live?
5. What action can be taken if it was considered harmful to return Lorna to Mona, or Neil?
6. What difference would it make if Lorna was 17?

Solutions

1. Because Lorna is voluntarily accommodated, the local authority does not have parental responsibility. This means that, subject to certain exceptions (*see* 2 below), and because she is under 16, anyone with parental responsibility (ie Mona) can remove her at any time without giving any notice, but only if he or she is willing or able to provide accommodation, or make arrangements for this.
2. Since anyone with parental responsibility can remove Lorna, Neil as her divorced father, can take her home. He would not have the right to do this, however, if a residence order had been granted to Mona and she wanted Lorna to stay with Mr and Mrs Bhutta. Court proceedings would then be necessary to settle the dispute (eg Neil or Lorna could apply for a residence order to be granted). Alternatively Neil may be able to persuade the local authority to place Lorna with him under their various accommodation duties.

If Neil and Mona had never married then, as an unmarried father, Neil's request could be ignored unless he had acquired parental responsibility in one of the ways permitted by the Children Act.

3. Before providing accommodation a local authority has a qualified duty to ascertain a child's wishes and give them due consideration, having regard to her age and understanding. A similar duty of consultation arises before any decision (such as to return Lorna to her mother) is made in respect of a child who is being looked after (the phrase 'looked after' includes a child voluntarily accommodated). Hence Lorna does have a right – albeit qualified – to be consulted.

4. Before making a decision about a child they are looking after the local authority must consult a range of people including 'any person whose wishes and feelings the authority consider to be relevant'. Guidance Vol. 3, para. 2.51 suggests consulting both the district health authority and the child's GP. Lorna's GP could therefore be consulted as could hospital staff.

5. Where Lorna's removal was considered harmful it may be possible to prevent it by obtaining an emergency protection order, interim care order or police protection. Alternatively where there is no time to take such action it may be possible to stop Lorna's removal by relying on Section 3(5) which empowers persons without parental responsibility 'to do what is reasonable in all the circumstances of the case for safeguarding or promoting a child's welfare'.

6. If Lorna was 17 and had been provided with accommodation then she would have an independent right to remain there (ie with Mr and Mrs Bhutta) despite parental opposition.

6

Organizational Framework of the Public Care System

The main source for this chapter is the Department of Health guidance document *Working together under the Children Act: a guide to arrangements for inter-agency co-operation for the protection of children from abuse*, HMSO, 1991.

The chapter looks at the organizational framework of the public care system (statutory and otherwise) and the investigative process. Although a number of different agencies are involved, notably social services departments, the police, NSPCC, the education service and voluntary organizations, the main focus will be on the distinctive role of health professionals and guardians ad litem.

Although the Children Act 1989 provides a new statutory code for the care and protection of children which is designed to promote and encourage inter-agency co-operation, it contains no guidance on how the different agencies should co-ordinate action, communicate information and develop effective policy and practice. Nevertheless, over the last 20 years various inter-agency mechanisms and procedures have evolved in response to a series of government reports and circulars (circulars, like guidance documents, are not in themselves law but are very persuasive statements of 'good practice'). These have attempted to establish a framework within which all the relevant agencies can carry out their responsibilities and develop and formalize inter-professional, multidisciplinary working practices. The current framework consists of three principal structures: Area Child Protection Committees; Child Protection Registers; and Child Protection Conferences.

Area Child Protection Committee

The Area Child Protection Committee (ACPC) has overall responsibility for co-ordinating current practice and developing, monitoring and reviewing child care policy within a particular area. Specific tasks include establishing, maintaining and reviewing local guidelines on procedures to be followed in individual cases (local procedural handbooks are issued to hospitals, schools etc); monitoring the implementation of legal procedures; and scrutinizing arrangements for inter-agency liaison and training. Each individual agency is responsible for co-ordinating policy and practice among its own personnel, although they should be based on the principles laid down by the ACPC. The committee comprises senior representatives of all the key agencies.

PRACTICE NOTES

Membership of the committee should include senior officers or professionals from the health authority, family health services authority and NHS Trusts (where appropriate).

Health professionals may be asked to contribute to the local ACPC's development and review of existing policy and practice.

Child Protection Register

The Child Protection Register (CPR) is a central record of all children who are considered by a relevant agency to be at risk. The register has no statutory basis or legal force. Nor is it a register of children who have been abused. It operates rather as a management tool which professionals can use as a speedy reference point when they are concerned about a child and want to check whether a protection plan already exists. Detailed guidance on the operation and management of the register is contained in *Working together* (Part 6). For registration purposes there are four categories of 'risk', namely neglect, physical injury, sexual abuse and emotional abuse. Registration is an important step, usually sanctioned by a case conference (*see* below). It should be formally reviewed every six months.

PRACTICE NOTES

Health professionals may be involved in various aspects of the registration process, notably:

- assessing whether the requirements for registration are met
- ensuring that multiple abuse registration is avoided (which can undermine the statistical value of the register and distort the protection plan) by advising on the appropriate category of registration
- assessing whether the criteria for de-registration have been met.

Child Protection Conference

The Child Protection Conference (CPC) commonly referred to as a 'case conference' is central to child protection procedures. It brings together the family and professionals and provides an opportunity to gather, evaluate, and exchange relevant information and agree a particular course of action. There are two kinds of CPCs – the initial CPC and the child protection review. The primary role of the initial CPC is to decide whether to register a child and agree a plan, whereas the main purpose of the child protection review is to review arrangements for the protection of the child, examine the current level of risk and consider whether inter-agency co-ordination is functioning effectively. Detailed guidance on the function, organization, attendance and chairing of conferences is provided in *Working together* (Part 6).

Specific recommendations are made to encourage and promote the active participation of children, their parents and other carers, reflecting the new emphasis on partnership. These include detailed practical suggestions to facilitate attendance and communication. In addition, ACPCs are urged to formally agree the principle of including parents and children in all conferences. In some cases, however, it is acknowledged that it may not be right to invite one or other parent to a conference, either in whole or in part. Their exclusion might be justified, for example, where there is supporting evidence of a strong risk of violence towards the professionals concerned or the child.

PRACTICE NOTES

A health professional may ask for a CPC to be convened when he or she believes the child is not adequately protected or when there is a need for a change to the child protection plan.

Health professionals may be asked to attend conferences or to submit written reports and appropriate records, such as growth charts.

Inter-agency co-operation

Although local authorities have the primary statutory responsibility for the investigation and prevention of child abuse and neglect it has long been recognized that protecting children usually involves and professionally concerns other agencies. However, the failure of different agencies to work effectively together has been identified as a major weakness in virtually every inquiry into child abuse in the last 20 years. Strengthening inter-agency co-operation was therefore seen as one of the main priorities and in 1988 the first version of the Department of Health's guidance, *Working together*, on interdisciplinary working was published to coincide with the Cleveland Report.

The original guidance needed to be revised, however, to take into account the requirements of the Children Act and to encourage a move away from the multi-agency approach where each agency operates within its own procedures, terminology, priorities, and resources, to a more integrated and co-ordinated inter-agency approach.

Overall, *Working together* seeks to establish a voluntary framework for inter-professional co-operation and communication at both operational and managerial levels. It not only includes detailed guidance on how individual cases should be handled but also on the development of joint agency and management policies. Important too, is the section it devotes to identifying the roles of various agencies and how their respective duties and functions should be organized (Part 4).

Predictably, health professionals are singled out as major contributors to the inter-agency care and protection of children and the following is a summary of paras. 4.18 to 4.33.

PRACTICE NOTES

Designated Senior Professionals (DSP). Each authority should identify a senior doctor, a senior nurse with a health visiting qualification and a senior midwife (designated senior professionals) to act as co-ordinator of all aspects of child protection work within their district. This includes:

- providing advice to social services departments and health professionals
- taking responsibility for identifying the training needs of their professional groups in child protection procedures (*see* Appendix 9 for further details of the DSP's role).

Midwives and health visitors. Contact with families during pregnancy, birth and the early care of children provides opportunities not just for the preparation and support of parents but also for initial assessments of the child's home environment and the quality of care currently, or likely, to be given. Any concerns, such as the need for a protection plan or a pre-birth child protection conference, should then be referred to the social services department.

All hospital staff. Hospital staff are expected:

- to be alert to indications of abuse and to carers who shop around for medical services in order to conceal the repeated nature of a child's injuries
- to be familiar with local procedures for checking the CPR and seek advice and assistance on procedural matters from the designated senior professional and on clinical issues from the appropriate specialist
- notify the health visitor or school nurse (and GP) of all visits made by children aged 0–16 years to the accident and emergency departments.

Primary and community health services. Domiciliary visits are recommended in situations 'where this is judged helpful to the family', for example travelling families, those in temporary accommodation, and especially those who do not readily take up the services offered. Professionals are advised to be aware of the signs and symptoms of abuse, and the procedures to follow.

Child and adolescent mental health services. Professionals who suspect abuse are expected to be fully conversant with local child protection procedures and able to focus on the needs of children and parents when they are asked to assess and/or treat families in which abuse is an issue.

If they are involved in assessing and treating an abuser then liaison with the Adult Psychiatric Service (and other relevant services) may also be necessary.

General practitioners. The role of GPs is said to be 'vital', especially in identifying at an early stage family stress which may point to risk of child abuse; noticing indications of significant harm, or likelihood of significant harm; contributing to child protection conferences and long-term support of the child and family.

Whenever they suspect abuse or that a child is at risk they are therefore urged to share information with appropriate statutory services and, if necessary, to discuss cases with colleagues.

They should also ensure that practice nurses receive training in the recognition of abuse and the operation of local procedures and have clearly defined professional support and clinical supervision.

Family health service authorities. These authorities should keep their contractors informed about child protection matters. In particular they should:

- identify a named person to co-ordinate the provision of advice to social service departments and to advise contractors
- ensure and monitor the suitability of local arrangements
- encourage the training of GPs in child protection work.

Private health care. Professionals are reminded that they also have duties to protect children and hence should be aware of relevant child protection procedures if they become suspicious about a child's care.

Guardians ad litem

A guardian ad litem (GAL) is normally an independent social worker selected from a panel established and administered by local authorities. The Act (Section 41) requires a GAL to be appointed in nearly all public law cases – a reform which could considerably increase their influence and the demand for their services.

The role of GALs is essentially proactive and protective. They are not supposed to be just advocates for the child in court but are expected to safeguard and represent the child's interests. The precise duties of a GAL are set out in rules of court. They include:

- appointing and instructing a solicitor to act for the child
- giving such advice to the child as is appropriate having regard to his or her age and understanding
- preparing a written report advising on the interests of the child
- making such investigations as may be necessary.

In addition the GAL has to advise the court on a number of matters, such as the child's wishes, options available in respect of the child and the timing of and appropriate forum for the proceedings.

PRACTICE NOTES

GALs are an important link between the court, the child and the various agencies involved in a case, and health professionals are most likely to be called upon to assist them in the following areas:

- *Advice to court* (medical or psychiatric examinations or assessments). GALs must advise the court whether the child is of sufficient understanding to consent to (or refuse) medical or psychiatric examination or other assessment that the court has power to require, direct or order.
- *Investigations*. Detailed investigations may require a GAL to contact and interview a wide range of people including any health professionals who may have been involved in the child's care or have information about the child and his or her family. Specialist medical advice may also be necessary in the course of enquiries.
- *Access to records*. Although GALs are entitled to examine and take copies of all social work records and files, as well as those of NSPCC and others, they have no legal right of access to health authority records, except in so far as they form part of the local authority's records.

Advising a GAL as to a child's understanding is a complex and demanding process which may require specialist knowledge, particularly if a child has communication problems.

The investigation process

Unlike most states in the USA where the law provides for compulsory reporting, local authorities have no statutory obligation to report suspected cases of child abuse or neglect. Nevertheless, they are required to investigate a child's welfare in a number of circumstances. Much of the law in this context repeats previous legislation but some changes have been made, notably responsibilities are now wider and more specific and include a positive obligation to investigate and conduct enquiries.

Section 47 is the principal governing provision. It is a complex section but basically imposes three main duties on local authorities. These are in addition to the investigative duties which may arise in the course of family proceedings, such as divorce and in cases where an education supervision order has not succeeded. The duties are as follows:

I. To initiate investigations and make enquiries
Local authorities must make enquiries whenever a child is at risk and subject to an emergency protection order, in police protection or where there is reasonable cause to suspect significant harm (or its likelihood).

2. *To focus enquiries*

Although the purpose and focus of the enquiries differs slightly depending on who has taken protective measures and where the child is currently living, the overall intention is twofold. First, the local authority must consider what powers it should exercise. For example, it may provide accommodation or another service or initiate care or supervision proceedings. Secondly, there is a new qualified duty to see the child if necessary.

3. *To take action following enquiries*

Local authorities now have a positive duty to take follow-up action. In cases where access to or information about a child is denied, compulsory measures must be initiated. In other cases, where no compulsory action is considered appropriate, they must consider whether the case should be reviewed. If it should, a date for the review must be fixed.

Inter-agency co-operation

The remaining provisions in Section 47 are aimed at promoting inter-agency co-operation. They require a wide range of agencies such as education, housing and health authorities to assist the local authority with their enquiries, in particular by providing relevant information and advice if called upon by the local authority to do so. Similar co-operative duties can be extended to other bodies and individuals by the Secretary of State.

Surprisingly, the list of agencies who are required to co-operate does not include the police or the probation service. These omissions were explained on the basis that 'police refusal to co-operate on any matter would be indefensible' and that probation officers, as officers of the court 'are already under a duty to assist in these matters'.

However, the obligation to co-operate is only a qualified duty, it does not oblige any person to assist a local authority 'where doing so would be unreasonable in all the circumstances of the case' (*see* Section 47(10)). Furthermore, no guidance is given in the Act about how agencies are expected to respond to the new statutory duty. Instead, arrangements for co-operation in the investigative process are contained in the guidance document *Working together* (Part 5). This outlines how individual cases should be dealt with and states that the investigative process under Section 47 comprises four prime tasks:

- to establish the facts about the circumstances giving rise to concern
- to decide if there are grounds for concern
- to identify sources and levels of risk
- to decide protective or other action in relation to the child and any others.

PRACTICE NOTES

Collaboration and co-operation in the investigative process may require health professionals to:

1. *Make referrals.* According to para. 5.11.1 of *Working together* the starting point of the investigative process is that any person, including health professionals, who has knowledge of, or a suspicion that a child is suffering significant harm, or is at risk of suffering harm, should refer their concerns to the appropriate agency. Referrals should be made in writing and should include as much factual information as is necessary.

2. *Exchange information.* Paras. 3.10–11 of *Working together* state:

> 'Arrangements for the protection of children can only be successful if all professional staff share and exchange information. . . . Ethical and statutory codes concerned with confidentiality and data protection are not intended to prevent the exchange of information between different professional staff who have a responsibility for ensuring the protection of children'.

See further *UKCC advisory paper for nursing, midwifery and health visiting* which advises practitioners to discuss matters fully with other practitioners and, if appropriate, a professional organization. They should also be prepared to justify their decision to pass on or withhold confidential information. *See* also the advice given by the British Medical Association that the interests of the child are paramount and override the general rule of professional confidence.

3. *Comply with local inter-agency guidelines.* Local procedural handbooks produced by the ACPC provide detailed guidance on the investigative process. In particular, health professionals may be asked to attend or report to the child protection conference, check records of the child and the family, be interviewed and contribute to the assessment of the child.

7

Compulsory Intervention

The Children Act completely recasts and restructures the law of care and supervision. Under previous legislation there were no less than 20 different routes into care, and many were based on different criteria. These are now replaced by one single composite ground, which applies to both care and supervision proceedings. The central importance of the new ground cannot be overestimated as it is now the only procedure through which compulsory long-term intervention can be triggered (wardship as a route into care has been removed by the Act). Note too, that care orders can no longer be used as a 'sentence' in criminal proceedings nor in 'truancy' cases.

Detailed guidance on how the new law should be applied and interpreted are contained in Guidance Volume 1 Court Orders (all references in this chapter are to this volume).

Before looking in more detail at the new ground it is important to stress that the Act gives the court considerable discretion as to whether or not to sanction coercive action. It must be satisfied that compulsory measures are necessary and that all other options, notably voluntary service provision under Part III of the Act, are inappropriate. As the guidance stresses:

'no decision to initiate care proceedings should be taken without clear evidence that provision of services for the child and his family (which may include accommodation voluntarily arranged) has failed or would be likely to fail to meet the child's needs adequately and that there is no suitable person prepared to apply to take over care of the child.' (para. 3.10)

PRACTICE NOTES

Health professionals may be asked to attend (or report to) the case conference which should always be convened whenever a possible care order case is identified (*see* para. 3.10).

Health professional advice may be essential in deciding the level and range of service provision which could 'retrieve the situation' and avoid the need for compulsory intervention.

In all cases where health professionals are uncertain about their role, eg in relation to other authorities or the courts, legal advice should be sought.

Care orders

A care order entitles a local authority to take over the care of a child possibly for good. It will normally involve the removal of the child from home because the authority considers it needs to have effective parental control.

Grounds for a care order: the 'threshold conditions'

The new grounds for a care order are set out in Section 31(2). They are:

(a) that the child concerned is suffering, or is likely to suffer significant harm; and
(b) that the harm or likelihood of harm is attributable to:
   I) the care given to the child, or likely to be given to him if the order were not made, not being what it would be reasonable to expect a parent to give him; or
   II) the child's being beyond parental control.

There is no power to make an order in respect of a child who is over 17, or 16 if married. These grounds are sometimes called the 'threshold conditions' or criteria. In the words of the Lord Chancellor they are

'the minimum circumstances which should always be found to exist before it can ever be justified for a court even to begin to contemplate whether the state should be able to intervene in family life'.

This means that they are not intended to be in themselves sufficient reason for making a care order and the court does not have to make an order just because the relevant criteria have been met. It must also apply the Section 1 principles, namely that the child's welfare is the paramount consideration, the no-delay principle, the non-intervention principle and the welfare check list.

Some of the terms used in the Act are defined by the Act (or require further explanation). For example:

Harm (Section 31(9))

Harm means ill-treatment or the impairment of health or development:

- development means physical, intellectual, emotional, social or behavioural development
- health means physical or mental health
- ill-treatment includes sexual abuse and forms of ill-treatment which are not physical.

Note in particular that:

- the definitions of harm are alternatives, therefore only one needs to be satisfied
- there is no specific reference to physical (or emotional) abuse in the definition of ill-treatment but these are included by implication

- ill-treatment is sufficient harm in itself whether or not it results in damage to the child's health or development
- abuse, whether sexual, physical or emotional, is not defined
- impairment of health or development seems wide enough to cover any case of neglect, such as poor nutrition, low standards of hygiene, poor emotional care or failure to seek treatment for an illness or condition.

Significant (Section 31(10))

In contrast to the expansive definition of 'harm', the word 'significant' is not defined. The only statutory guidance is contained in Section 31(10). This provides that where the facts relate to health or development, as opposed to ill-treatment, the child's health and development must be compared with that which could be reasonably expected of a 'similar' child. Points to stress here are:

1. According to the guidance (paras. 3.19–21) the word 'significant' should be given its dictionary definition of 'considerable, noteworthy or important' and should exclude minor shortcomings in health care or minor deficits in physical, psychological or social development unless cumulatively they are having, or are likely to have, serious or lasting effects upon the child.
2. The decision as to whether harm is or is not significant is essentially one of fact and is for the court to decide.
3. Significance can relate to the seriousness of the harm or the implications of it. For example, a broken leg or fractured skull would be serious injuries in themselves but a cigarette burn or throwing a child, even if they did not cause an injury, could have far greater implications.
4. Comparison with a hypothetical 'similar child' (only necessary in cases of impairment of health and development) involves comparison with a child of the same age and with similar special characteristics or needs, for example arising from a disability. So a six-year-old deaf child must be compared with another hypothetical six-year-old deaf child.
5. The extent to which social, environmental and cultural factors should be considered when making comparisons is unclear.
6. Once the comparison is made between the hypothetical similar child and the child in question the court must decide whether the degree of disparity is significant.

'Is suffering' or 'is likely to suffer'

Care proceedings can be based either on actual (current) or likely (future) harm. The word 'likely' is not defined but the guidance (para. 3.22) gives the following examples of when the 'likely' ground might apply: where a child has suffered significant harm in the past and is likely to do so again because of some recurring circumstance; to protect a child who has not yet been harmed but who is at risk because of family history; and to prevent parents removing a child from voluntary accommodation to an unsuitable home environment.

The court has said (*see* London Borough of Newham v. AG (1992)2 FCR 119) that the phrase 'likely' does not mean that the court must be satisfied on the balance of probabilities that there was a likelihood of harm. In looking to the future the court has to assess the risk and should not be asked to perform a strict legalistic analysis of the words used in the Act.

Reasonable parental care

Once significant harm or its likelihood has been proved, only one further element of the threshold criteria needs to be satisfied, which is that the harm is attributable to lack of reasonable parental care or the child being beyond parental control (*see* below). There are two strands to this element of the criteria. Firstly there has to be a link but no direct causation. Secondly, the court must ask itself 'What kind of care would a hypothetical reasonable parent provide for the child in question taking into account any special characteristics or needs he or she may have?' Having decided what that standard is the court must then consider how the child's actual or likely care measures up. Points to note here are:

- the word 'care' is not defined in the Act but is expected to be broadly interpreted, especially as the guidance states that it 'must mean providing for the child's health and total development (physical, intellectual, emotional, social and behavioural) and not just having physical charge of him'
- the approach taken by the court is both objective (it looks at what a 'reasonable' parent would do) and subjective (it considers any special characteristics the child may have)
- some children may need a higher standard of care than others because they have complex special needs, and a reasonable parent is expected to meet them
- orders can be obtained in cases where both the harm and parental failure is anticipated rather than currently occurring
- harm caused solely by a third party is excluded (unless the parent has failed to prevent it).

Beyond parental control

According to the guidance (para. 3.25) this covers cases where whatever the standard of care available, the child is not benefiting from it because of lack of parental control. This ground existed in previous legislation, although in the past it was not linked with harm to the child as it now is.

PRACTICE NOTES

Health professionals may be asked:

- whether the harm is 'significant'
- about the appropriate choice of comparators and what standard of health and development it would be reasonable to expect in a child with 'similar' attributes

- to assess the risk of a child suffering significant harm in the future
- to determine whether the harm is attributable to parental failure or has another cause
- to advise on the appropriate standard of care which could reasonably be expected of 'reasonable parents', especially when a child's health needs are complex, since this may require a higher standard of care than is normally necessary.

Effect of a care order

Under the old law the legal effect of a care order was uncertain and confusing. Now, because there is only one route into care, the respective rights, powers and responsibilities of parents and local authorities are much clearer. Provisions governing access to (ie contact with) children in care have also been substantially reformed. Similarly, new rules have been introduced to control the return home 'on trial' of children who are still subject to a care order.

Parental responsibility

Section 33(1) states that once a care order is made the local authority has a duty to receive the child into its care and keep him or her there as long as the order remains in force. It lasts until the child reaches 18 unless it is brought to an end sooner. This provision provides the legal foundation for a local authority's responsibilities and also establishes a broad framework within which decisions about upbringing can be made.

A care order gives the local authority parental responsibility which it shares with those who already have it (usually the child's parents) However, this 'sharing' arrangement does not mean that everybody with parental responsibility has an equal say on matters of upbringing since the Act clearly gives the local authority the 'upper hand' should disputes arise. It does this by virtue of a seemingly unimportant sub-section (Section 33(3)(b)) in which it states that a local authority has the power to limit (and thereby control) how others exercise their parental responsibility, although this must only be done when 'necessary to safeguard and promote the child's welfare'. Nor does it prevent a parent who is physically caring for the child, on a weekend visit for example, from doing what is 'reasonable in all the circumstances of the case to safeguard and promote the child's welfare'.

However, local authorities do not have a completely 'free hand' in matters of upbringing. First the Act prescribes the way they should look after children (*see* Chapter 9). Secondly, local authorities cannot change the child's religion, appoint a guardian or consent to adoption. Furthermore, a change in the child's surname or its removal from the United Kingdom for more than a month requires the written consent of all those with parental responsibility or a court order.

PRACTICE NOTES

Health professionals may be involved in disputes about the exercise of parental responsibility, especially those which focus on health-related aspects of upbringing.

Contact

Access to children in care has long been controversial and although major reforms were introduced a decade ago, giving parents greater rights to challenge access arrangements, these largely failed to bring about the expected improvements. Accordingly the Act has introduced additional reforms which are governed both by Section 34 and regulations (*see* the Contact with Children Regulations 1991 and Vol. 3, Chapter 6). The effect of these is that local authorities must allow reasonable contact with a child in care to parents (including an unmarried father even if he has not got parental responsibility), guardians, those who had a residence order when the care order was made, and those who had care of the child as a result of wardship, unless directed otherwise by a court.

The phrase 'reasonable contact' is not defined in the Act but is expected to be interpreted broadly and to include not just personal meetings and visits but also other means of keeping the family bonds alive such as letters, telephone calls and an exchange of photographs.

In addition the following features of the new provision governing 'care contact orders' should be noted:

- contact arrangements can be controlled by the courts and parents, children and others have increased rights to challenge existing arrangements
- in emergencies a local authority can refuse contact for up to seven days without getting the court's prior permission
- if a local authority (or the child concerned) wants to stop contact for longer than seven days, they must apply to the court
- detailed regulations govern procedures for refusing contact and varying or suspending existing arrangements
- the court can make care contact orders (with or without conditions) either in response to an application or on its own initiative
- the court must consider proposed contact arrangements before a care order is made and invite the parties to comment on them
- contact orders can be varied and discharged and made either at the same time as the care order itself or later.

PRACTICE NOTES

Health professionals need to be aware of the presumption of reasonable contact and make appropriate arrangements, especially when a child is in hospital and is visited by a parent or other person entitled to contact.

Health professionals may be involved when questions about suspension, restriction, refusal or supervision of contact arise.

Professional expertise may be essential in communicating decisions about contact to parents and children, especially those with communication difficulties.

Placement with parents

Even though a care order is in force, it may be appropriate (and has been common practice for some time) to allow a child to return home on a 'trial' basis. Such arrangements are now controlled by a new set of regulations (Placement of Children with Parents regulations 1991). These have three broad aims: to provide a framework for 'good professional practice'; to achieve a better balance between the rehabilitative and protective functions of local authorities; and to ensure that any trial period is closely regulated and monitored.

The regulations require that extensive enquiries have to be made about a child's health, social and educational needs and the suitability of both the accommodation and various members of the household before he or she is returned home for more than 24 hours (*see* Vol. 3, Chapter 5 for further details).

PRACTICE NOTES

Health professionals may be involved in the following areas:

1. *Enquiries about carers.* Enquiries may necessitate medical examinations and reports into the suitability (ie health and personality) of the proposed carers and other household members (Regulation 3).

2. *Assessment of the child.* A medical assessment may be necessary to assess whether a home placement is practicable.

3. *Agreements.* Agreements should be reached on a variety of matters including the child's health and need for health care and surveillance (Regulation 7).

4. *Support and supervision of the placement.* Placements must be supervised and appropriate support given, especially when a child has complex needs or a disability (Regulation 9).

5. *Notification.* The district health authority (for the district in which the child is living) and the child's GP must be notified of the placement decision (Regulation 8).

Interim care orders

An interim care order is a short-term 'holding' order often used to keep a child in care after the expiry of emergency procedures or as a prelude to a full care order. Although temporary, it can involve substantial intervention in a child's life and the reforms introduced here have two broad aims: to enable the child to be suitably protected whilst proceedings are progressing, and to see that interim measures operate only for as long as is necessary.

Interim orders can be made when the court adjourns proceedings for a full care or supervision order, or directs the local authority to investigate the child's circumstances as in family proceedings such as divorce. In either case the court must be satisfied 'that there are reasonable grounds for believing' that the child's circumstances fulfil the criteria for a full care order (Section 38). Note that this is a 'lower test' than that needed for a full care order, where proof of significant harm or its likelihood is required. In addition, the welfare principle, the welfare check list, the non-intervention and no-delay principles must be considered.

An interim order generally has the same legal effect as a full care order. This means that the local authority acquire, and share, parental responsibility and the provisions about contact and home placements apply (*see* above). However, there are two major differences between full and interim care orders. First, the court determines the duration of the interim order which can initially be made for eight weeks with extensions of up to four weeks. Secondly, the court now has extensive powers to control medical and psychiatric examinations and assessments.

Medical or psychiatric examinations and assessments

When the court thinks it appropriate, court directions can be given about medical or psychiatric examination or other assessment of the child. Such directions may be essential, as where medical evidence is obtained during proceedings without the court's permission, the court can refuse to consider it. Note in particular the following aspects of the courts' powers:

- the word 'assessment' is not defined but guidance is given in *Working together under the Children Act 1991* (*see* above) and *Protecting children: a guide for social workers undertaking a comprehensive assessment*, HMSO, 1991
- the court can prohibit examinations or assessments altogether or make them subject to its specific approval
- directions can be given either when the interim order is first made or at any time whilst it is in force
- all directions can be varied
- children under 16 who are of sufficient understanding to make an informed decision (they are 'Gillick competent') can refuse to submit to an examination or assessment
- competent children over 16 can also refuse their consent
- the court can determine the type of examination or assessment and by whom it should be carried out (an AIDS test has been ordered under this provision).

PRACTICE NOTES

'Local inter-agency arrangements should aim to establish a pool of health and other professionals as trained experts who may be called upon to participate in a wide-ranging programme of multidisciplinary assessments and examinations' (Vol. I, para. 3.48).

Health professionals may be asked to advise on the nature, scope and objective of examinations and assessments and the detailed directions that should be specified.
Before examining or assessing a child, health professionals should ascertain:

- who has parental responsibility
- who has the right to consent − court directions do not override the right of 'Gillick competent' children under 16 (or those aged 16 and over) to refuse to submit to such examinations or assessments
- whether specific directions have been given
- whether the examination or assessment is to be used in court proceedings.

Health professionals should comply with any specified directions or consider whether a variation should be sought. A parent who objects to a child's examination or assessment can seek a direction from the court.

Supervision orders

A supervision order places a child (under 17, or 16 if married) under the supervision of a local authority or probation officer. It is used when a court decides that a close eye needs to be kept on a child in order to monitor his or her care, for example whilst parenting skills are improved. Although a supervision order is compulsory it is less drastic and disruptive than a care order: the child remains at home and parental responsibility is not acquired by the local authority. Most of the reforms introduced by the Act are designed to make supervision orders more effective and thus more popular.

Grounds for a supervision order: the 'threshold conditions'

The grounds for making a supervision order are identical to those for a care order, ie the child must have suffered or is likely to suffer significant harm. Similarly the Section 1 principles must be applied (the paramountcy of the child's welfare, the welfare check list and the non-intervention and no-delay principles). This means that the court has a wide discretion as to whether to make an order, especially as the Act gives no guidance as to when a supervision order should be made rather than a care order.

Effects of a supervision order

These are spelt out in detail in Section 35 and Schedule 3. The most important new feature introduced by the Act is the increased powers given to supervisors to impose specific requirements on children and their carers. Changes have also been made to the order's duration. It can initially be made for one year with possible extensions, but the total duration cannot exceed three years and it ends automatically when the child is 18.
The supervisor's duties are to 'advise, assist and befriend the child'; take such steps as are reasonably necessary to give effect to the order; and consider whether

to apply for a variation or discharge of the order where it is not being wholly complied with or is no longer necessary.

Requirements can be imposed on the supervised child or 'responsible person'. They may, for example, require the child to live in a specified place or participate in specified activities. Additional requirements can also be imposed on the 'responsible person' (ie anyone with parental responsibility or with whom the child is living). There are also detailed provisions governing health care.

Health requirements

When a supervision order is made medical and psychiatric examinations and treatment may be necessary and the court has extensive powers to impose a wide range of health-related requirements. Virtually all these provisions existed in previous legislation.

1. *Psychiatric and medical examinations* (Schedule 3 para. 4). Directions about medical or psychiatric examinations can be made which may, for example, specify that the child should be examined from 'time to time as directed by the supervisor'. In addition, the order may name who is to carry out the examination and should specify where it is to take place. The child can only be required to be a resident patient at a health service hospital, or in the case of a psychiatric examination, at a hospital or mental nursing home, if the court is satisfied by medical evidence that the child requires and may be susceptible to treatment, and that a period as a resident patient is necessary.

No directions can be imposed on a competent young person of 16 or over, or a 'Gillick competent' child under 16 unless the child consents and satisfactory arrangements have been, or can be, made for the examination.

2. *Psychiatric and medical treatment* (Schedule 3 para. 5). Directions about psychiatric and medical treatment can only be included if the court is satisfied, on the advice of practitioners approved for the purposes of Section 12 of the Mental Health Act 1983, that the child's condition requires and may be susceptible to treatment. In psychiatric cases the court must also be satisfied that the child's condition does not warrant detention under the Mental Health Act 1983. The treatment must be carried out by, or under the direction of, a registered medical practitioner who may be named.

In addition the order must specify what treatment is to be provided; how long it is to last; and where it is to be carried out (the child may be a non-resident or resident patient in a national health service hospital or, in psychiatric cases, in a hospital or mental nursing home).

As with examinations, competent young people of 16 and over and 'Gillick competent' under-16-year-olds must consent and satisfactory arrangements must be made available.

3. *Changes to treatment.* In some cases specified treatment may need to be changed. A written report must be submitted to the child's supervisor by the medical practitioner if he or she is unwilling to continue such treatment or considers it needs changing because:

• it should extend beyond the period originally specified
• the child needs different treatment

- the child is no longer susceptible to treatment; or
- the child does not require it anymore.

The supervisor must then refer this report to the court, which may cancel or vary its requirements.

PRACTICE NOTES

Health professionals may be asked to advise the court on the need, nature and scope of appropriate examinations, assessments and treatment. Before conducting such procedures health professionals should ascertain:

- who has parental responsibility
- who has the right to consent – health-related requirements do not override the rights of competent young people (whether over or under 16) to refuse to submit to them.

When carrying out examinations, assessments or treatment, health professionals must comply with any specified health-related requirements. Health professionals should also be aware of the need to submit a report to the supervisor if treatment requirements change.

Interim supervision orders

Under previous legislation there was no power to make an interim supervision order. This anomaly has now been remedied and one can now be made whenever the court adjourns proceedings for a full care or supervision order, or directs the local authority to investigate a child's circumstances (in family proceedings such as divorce). In addition, an interim supervision order must also be made whenever a court makes a residence order in care or supervision proceedings, unless it is satisfied that the child's welfare can be satisfactorily safeguarded without one.

Interim supervision orders are governed by Section 38 which also governs interim care orders (*see* above). Accordingly, the provisions regulating the order's duration and the court's powers to give directions about medical and psychiatric examinations and assessments also apply.

An interim order generally has the same effect as a full supervision order, but its duration is different and the court's extensive powers to control medical and psychiatric examinations and treatment contained in paragraphs 4 and 5 of Schedule 3 do not apply.

PRACTICE NOTES

As with interim care orders health professionals may be asked to advise on the need, scope and objective of examinations and assessments and the detailed directions that should be specified etc (*see* Practice notes on interim care orders, pages 80–1).

Procedural aspects of care and supervision proceedings

The Act and accompanying rules of court contain detailed procedural and jurisdictional provisions. The following are some of the most important aspects covered:

- *Who can apply for orders?* A local authority or authorized person (NSPCC).
- *Where are proceedings heard?* Usually they start in the magistrates' courts.
- *Who can participate in proceedings?* Participants include 'full' parties such as the applicants, those with parental responsibility and the child, also those who are not parties but to whom notice of the proceedings must be given (eg a child's current carers).
- *Are there rights of appeal?* All parties have full rights of appeal against a magistrate's decision to make or refuse an order.
- *Can orders be discharged?* A care order can be brought to an end by adoption, a residence order, a supervision order or a successful discharge application. Supervision orders can be discharged by a care order or a successful discharge application.

Education supervision orders

A care order can no longer be obtained on educational grounds alone. Instead a new education supervision order is introduced to deal with truancy cases. According to Section 36 this order can only be made when a child is not being 'properly educated' (ie not receiving full-time education suitable to his age, ability and aptitude and any special educational needs he may have). In addition the court must apply the Section 1 principles, ie the paramountcy of the child's welfare; the non-intervention and no-delay principles and the welfare check list.

Despite the new order it is still possible to make a care or supervision order in non-school attendance cases, providing the threshold conditions in Section 31 are satisfied (*see* above).

PRACTICE NOTES

Health professionals may be required to contribute to the preparation of health-related aspects of the court report which must accompany any application for an education supervision order.

Case studies

Case study 12

May is eight years old. She was taken into care not long after her mother, Nina, started living with her current boyfriend, a violent man with a string of convictions. At first May did not seem to be affected by Nina's new relationship but once her second child, Peter, was born the practice nurse at the local health centre began to suspect that May was being neglected. May's care further deteriorated when Nina began to suffer from postnatal depression and a neighbour reported often seeing May hungry and very dirty.

Despite the provision of a wide range of support services, care proceedings were eventually taken and May is currently living with foster parents. But now there is also concern over Peter who is nearly a year old, since his recent checkup revealed that his developmental progress was worryingly slow. Nina has discussed his care with the health visitor, Peggy, and admits that she finds it difficult to look after him, especially recently as she is expecting her third child in a few weeks and gets very tired.

Last week May was admitted to hospital following an accident in the school bus. Whilst there she is regularly visited by her grandfather, Owen, but after one such visit she seems very distressed but refuses to say why. When Owen turns up for his usual visit one afternoon, May hides under the bed covers and refuses to come out until Owen has gone. Owen says that as a member of May's family he is legally entitled to see her when he wants to.

1. On what grounds were care proceedings likely to have been taken in respect of May?
2. Were such proceedings inevitable once the threshold conditions were satisfied?
3. Has Owen got a right to see his granddaughter in hospital? Would the answer be different if it was May's father who was insisting on visiting rights?
4. How could May's father be stopped from visiting her and would hospital staff be involved in this process?
5. What action should Peggy, the health visitor, take in respect of Peter?
6. Are care proceedings based on the possibility of future harm possible in respect of Peter?

Solutions

1. Care proceedings are likely to have been based on May's health or development being impaired. In other words she satisfied the threshold criteria in Secton 31 in that she was suffering 'significant harm' attributable to the care given to her 'not being what it would be reasonable to expect a parent to give'. The word 'health' is widely defined in the Act as is the word 'development' and could therefore cover any case of neglect such as poor nutrition and low standards of hygiene.
2. Even though one of the threshold criteria in Section 31 was satisfied, a care order was not inevitable as a court would have had to consider the Act's fundamental principles, in particular, the non-intervention principle. Therefore it could have decided that in May's particular situation a care order was not appropriate because it was not the best way of promoting her welfare.

3. When a child is subject to a care order there is a statutory presumption that 'reasonable' contact will be allowed between the child and various people such as her parents, guardians and those with residence orders. This means that Owen has no right to see May unless he had a residence order immediately before the care order was made.

   However, May's father does have the right to reasonable contact whether or not he has parental responsibility, unless this has been restricted, terminated or otherwise regulated in ways permitted by Section 34 of the Children Act.

4. When a care order is in force a local authority can apply to court to stop contact. But when contact needs to be prevented 'as a matter of urgency to safeguard or promote' May's welfare it can be stopped for up to seven days without the court's permission.

   A child can refuse to see a person who visits and need not obtain an order to do so. However, if there is no other way of avoiding contact (which there might not be given that May's father wants contact) then an order may have to be obtained to stop contact, which either May or the local authority can apply for.

5. Peter is not in care but he may qualify as a child 'in need' and therefore be entitled to a range of services, for example day care provision, guidance, counselling or a family centre. Temporary accommodation may also be an option. Given the strong emphasis in the Act on avoiding compulsory action and protecting children by way of voluntary arrangements and partnership with parents, Peggy should contact social services so that a co-ordinated package of services can be planned and provided for Peter. Peggy should contribute to the assessment of Peter's needs, especially his health and developmental needs.

6. Yes, if voluntary arrangements do not work then care proceedings can be taken on the basis of the 'significant harm' that Peter is 'likely to suffer' in the future, which is attributable to the care 'likely to be given to him not being what it would be reasonable to expect a parent to give'. However, the non-intervention principle would again apply so the court would only make a care order if it was thought better than making no order at all.

Case study 13

Nigel is nine years old and the subject of an interim care order. When the order was made very detailed medical directions were included, not only naming Paula as the paediatrician who should carry out an examination and assessment but also specifying precisely what medical tests should be carried out.

An interim care order has also been made in respect of Nigel's sister, Olga, aged 13. Again, detailed medical directions were included in the order, and Paula was to conduct the examination. When the order was made Olga agreed to be examined, but just as Paula was about to start examining her she changed her mind.

1. Must Paula follow the court's directions and examine Olga against her wishes?
2. If Paula thinks that the court's directions about Nigel's examination are wrong can she do anything to get them changed?

3. If interim supervision orders had been made in respect of Nigel and Olga could the court have given detailed directions about medical examinations and assessments? If so, what rights would Olga have to refuse to submit to them and could medical directions in respect of Nigel be changed?

Solutions

1. Court directions authorizing examination and assessment do not absolve health professionals from their responsibility to satisfy themselves that a child of sufficient age and understanding does in fact consent. Paula should not therefore examine Olga if she is 'Gillick competent' and capable of an informed refusal. In practice, courts are extremely reluctant to give directions about a child's examination unless they have satisfied themselves that the health professional concerned has been consulted and is willing and able to carry out the required procedures.
2. Any party named in a court medical direction can apply to the court for it to be varied. Paula should therefore make the appropriate application to change tests ordered for Nigel.
3. As with interim care orders, medical examinations and assessments can be included in interim supervision orders. These can be varied on application by anyone named in the order (ie Paula). Children (possibly Olga) who are sufficiently mature to make an informed decision can refuse to submit to them.

8

Child Protection

This chapter considers Part V of the Act which radically reforms the law of child protection. New orders are created, notably the child assessment and emergency protection orders and substantial amendments are made to other protective measures such as the recovery order. Police powers and provisions governing the abduction of children in care and in 'safe' houses for runaway children are also restructured.

Child assessment order

The child assessment order (CAO) is a completely new order which had no parallel in previous legislation. Its main purpose is to enable a child to be seen so that enough can be found out about his or her health, development or treatment to decide what further action, if any, is required. The CAO is therefore not designed for emergency situations where the child is in immediate danger but is a lesser, heavily court-controlled order dealing with the narrow issue of examination and assessment. Official guidance suggests it should be used when there is 'serious concern' for a child's safety, but no hard evidence, and where the harm 'is long-term and cumulative rather than sudden and severe' (Vol. 1, para. 4.9).

The CAO is therefore ideal for resolving the classic (but not uncommon) dilemma faced if informal attempts to achieve an assessment of a child have failed but there is real concern, and insufficient evidence for such, about a child's health, development or safety. For example, unco-operative parents may have consistently resisted attempts to arrange an assessment by agreement or a child may suddenly have stopped attending a nursery or family centre in suspicious circumstances. Alternatively, neighbours may have reported repeated screaming.

Grounds for a child assessment order (Section 43)

A CAO can only be made if the court is satisfied that the applicant (a local authority or NSPCC) has reasonable cause to suspect that the child is suffering, or is likely to suffer, significant harm and an assessment is required to determine whether or not this is so, and it is unlikely that an assessment can be carried out without an order.

In addition the court must apply the welfare principle (but not the welfare check list) and the non-intervention and no-delay principles. As with all orders under the Act an order is not automatic just because the relevant conditions have been met.

Other features worth noting about the new order are:

- it does not allow an assessment of the family, only the individual child
- an application should always be preceded by an investigation under Section 47 (*see* Chapter 6) which should not be superficial
- arrangements for the assessment should be made before the court application is made
- the court is unlikely to make an order unless it is satisfied that all reasonable efforts have been made to persuade the child's carers to co-operate
- the court can treat an application for a CAO as though it were an application for an emergency protection order
- a CAO can be made at the same time as any of the Section 8 orders or an education supervision order.

Effects of a child assessment order

An order cannot last longer than seven days but need not begin immediately. It could, for example, be postponed until a hospital bed became available. However, because the order is not intended to be too interventionist it does not affect existing parental responsibility which is accordingly retained by whoever had it before the order was made. This means that unless the court has given permission the applicant cannot do anything without parental consent. The order also requires any person who is in a position to do so to produce the child and to comply with any specified directions. Where a medical or social history forms an essential part of the assessment, the order can also require that person to answer questions about the child.

The assessment

Not surprisingly the main effect of a CAO is to authorize an assessment of the child. Although the word 'assessment' is not defined in the Act, guidance on various types of assessment is provided in the Department of Health document *Protecting children: a guide to social workers undertaking a comprehensive assessment* (1988). Given the short time available, however, it is unlikely that anything more than an initial medical and social work assessment (and perhaps a psychiatric assessment) will be possible, although the court can give detailed directions about the kind of assessment and who should carry it out (*see* below).

As with similar provisions elsewhere in the Act (for example, interim care and supervision orders) the Act specifically states that 'Gillick competent' children under 16 of 'sufficient understanding to make an informed decision' can refuse to submit to a medical or psychiatric examination or other assessment. Competent children over 16 also have this right of informed refusal.

The child will usually stay at home whilst the order lasts. However, in exceptional circumstances he or she might be kept away from home, but only if the order specifically authorizes the child's removal. Examples when an overnight stay in hospital might be appropriate are given in the guidance and include where a child has an eating disorder, seriously disturbed sleep patterns or other symptoms which require 24-hour continuous monitoring (Vol. 1, para. 4.15).

Court directions: health examinations and assessments

The court has wide powers to include directions about the nature and objective of the assessment. Directions could, for example, specify that the assessment should be limited to a medical examination or cover other aspects of the child's health and development. It could direct where and by whom it should be carried out, perhaps naming the child's usual doctor or another health professional known to the family. In some cases the expertise of a specialist such as a paediatrician or psychiatrist may be necessary. The court can also specify how long the examination should take and what aids such as toys, dolls and writing instruments should be used. In addition, directions could specify how the examination should be recorded.

Action after a child assessment order

What happens if the child is not 'produced' or refuses to be assessed? Deliberate failure to comply with the order would probably be sufficient to warrant an emergency protection order or police protection (*see* below). But if a mature child refuses to be assessed the courts are not expected to change the child's mind. This is stressed in the guidance:

> 'professionals should take particular care to avoid coercing the child into agreement even where there is a belief that the refusal to comply is itself the product of coercion by a relative or friend' (Vol. 1, para. 4.13).

Otherwise, follow-up action will be determined by the result of the assessment and voluntary arrangements may be appropriate or possibly compulsory measures such as an interim care or supervision order or an emergency protection order.

PRACTICE NOTES

Health professionals have a key role to play in various aspects of the CAO, notably:

Investigations prior to the application. Investigations are expected: to be pursued on a multidisciplinary basis with pooling of information and consultation; and to be considered at a case conference convened under local child protection procedures (Vol. 1, para. 4.23).

Health professionals may thus be required to co-operate with the local authority in the investigative process by:

- contributing to the case conference (and any review)
- checking records
- exchanging information
- being interviewed.

Communication with parents. A CAO is unlikely to be granted unless the court is satisfied that reasonable efforts have been made to persuade the child's parents (or other carers) to co-operate with a voluntary assessment. They are therefore expected to be told that an order may be applied for as well as its legal effect and other detailed implications.

A familiar and trusted health professional may be the most appropriate person to talk to a child's carers, giving them reassurance and relevant information and persuading them to co-operate.

Communication with children. In assessing whether a child has sufficient understanding to refuse consent to an examination or assessment the guardian ad litem may need to seek the assistance of health professionals, particularly where the child suffers from a handicap which impairs his or her ability to communicate.

Planning the assessment. Given the order's short duration the guidance recommends that necessary arrangements should be made in advance of the application, to enable an initial multidisciplinary assessment of the child's medical, intellectual, emotional, social and behavioural needs to be completed satisfactorily in the time available (Vol. 1, para. 4.12).

Health professionals should therefore liaise with other appropriate agencies in planning in advance the matters to be covered during the assessment, the practical arrangements for carrying it out, and the best way to involve parents and minimize trauma for the child.

Medical examinations and assessments: court directions. The court may need to take professional advice about the type, nature and objective of the assessment and whether the child needs to be kept away from home.

Carrying out the assessment. According to the guidance, although there may be occasions when the most obvious need is for a medical assessment, an assessment should always have a multidisciplinary dimension as the difficulties and needs of children must always be seen in the context of their social needs and the abilities and limitations of their parents, extended family and local community to meet them.

All professional practitioners working with the family should be encouraged to contribute to a multidisciplinary assessment both to pool information and to make proposals for future action to support the family (Vol. 1, para. 4.25).

Before examining or assessing a child, health professionals should ascertain:

- who has parental responsibility
- who has the right to consent − court directions on examinations or assessments do not override the rights of mature children to refuse to submit to them
- whether specific directions have been given
- whether the assessment is to be used in court proceedings.

When carrying out the assessment health professionals should ensure that they comply with any specified directions or consider whether a variation should be sought.

Contact arrangements. When the child is kept away from home during the assessment health professionals should be aware of, and comply with, any specific directions which have been given in the order about contact between the child and his or her family.

Race and culture. Health professional advice may be necessary to ensure that racial and cultural factors are sensitively and appropriately considered, with regard to physical examination for example.

Emergency protection order

The emergency protection order (EPO) is a new order which replaces the much discredited place of safety order. Its purpose is to provide immediate short-term protection in 'genuine emergencies where the situation is sufficiently serious to justify severe powers of intervention'. Although the new order derives from previous legislation, nearly every aspect of it is new, including grounds for the order, its effect and duration.

Overall the reforms have three main aims: to promote decisive, speedy action when necessary; to provide parents, children and others with reasonable opportunities to present their points of view; and to ensure that emergency measures are not used prematurely as a routine response to allegations of child abuse or as a routine first step to initiating care proceedings.

Grounds for an emergency protection order (Section 44)

There are three separate grounds, but as with all other orders under the Act an order is not automatic just because the relevant criteria have been met. The court must also consider the welfare principle, non-intervention and no-delay principles, but not the welfare check list.

Ground 1: 'significant harm'

Under this ground an order can be made if significant harm is likely if the child is not removed to, or kept in, a safe place. Points to note are:

- 'significant harm' includes ill-treatment or impairment of health and development (*see* Section 31 in Chapter 7 for full definition)
- the harm need not be current as the ground specifically refers to future (likely) harm, for example, where a baby has just been born into a family with a long history of violent behaviour to young children or where a child is away from home but likely to be harmed if returned
- the majority of applications are likely to be made by local authorities or the NSPCC. In 'dire circumstances' anybody can act independently and apply for an order

- in deciding whether to grant an order the court will want to know precisely why urgent action is necessary and whether the child can be removed with the parents' co-operation
- the court can take into account any evidence and give as much weight to it as considered appropriate; this includes any relevant hearsay, opinions, health visiting or social work records and medical records (Section 45(7)).

PRACTICE NOTES

A health professional may in rare cases be the most appropriate person to apply for an order.

Grounds 2 and 3: frustrated access

The other two grounds both deal with the same kinds of cases where investigations into the child's circumstances are being obstructed. Either local authorities can apply when they are carrying out their investigative duties (under Section 47) and when access to the child, which is urgently required, is being unreasonably refused.

Alternatively, 'authorized persons' (ie the NSPCC) who are making enquiries about a child's welfare can apply in the same circumstances, except that they must also satisfy the court that they have reasonable cause to suspect that a child is suffering, or is likely to suffer, significant harm. Points to note here are:

- 'access' is not defined but it is assumed to involve face-to-face contact lasting for a reasonable length of time
- 'unreasonably refused' again is not defined but the guidance suggests (Vol. 1, para. 4.39) that refusal of a request to see a sleeping child in the middle of the night may not be unreasonable, but refusal to allow access at a reasonable time without good reason could well be
- whether or not access is urgently required is ultimately a question of fact which depends on the nature of the suspicion, the age of the child, and existing opportunities to see him or her
- the court can consider hearsay, health records etc (see Ground 1, page 92).

Effects of an emergency protection order

Under the old law the effects of an order – particularly the position concerning medical examinations and the rights of parents to challenge decisions and see their children – were unclear and frequently misunderstood. These uncertainties have been largely removed by the Act, notably by giving the court new powers to give directions (see below). Other new provisions aim to strengthen the force of orders and facilitate tracing children at risk. The main effects of an order are as follows:

1. It can last initially for up to eight days although the court can make a shorter order and it may be extended (once only) for a further seven days.

2. Any person who is in a position to do so must comply with the order and produce the child. The court can also authorize the applicant to enter and search premises (which can be backed up by a warrant authorizing police assistance).

3. An EPO also authorizes the child's removal or prevents his or her removal from current accommodation, such as a hospital, providing that the child's welfare requires such draconian action. Hence, if an applicant finds that the child is not likely to suffer harm because, for example, the suspected abuser has left, then the child should be left at home. Furthermore when a child is removed or detained the Act specifically provides that he or she should be returned or released once it is safe to do so.

4. Whoever obtains an EPO also acquires limited parental responsibility. It only lasts while the order is in force and only permits short-term decisions to be made which are 'reasonably required to safeguard and promote the child's welfare'. This means, for example, arranging the child's temporary accommodation.

PRACTICE NOTES

Medical assistance. To provide immediate medical aid or determine whether the child needs to be removed it may be necessary for a health professional to be present when an EPO is exercised. Accordingly an order can direct that a doctor, nurse or health visitor accompany social workers exercising any of their powers under the order (Section 45(12)).

Similarly, the court may direct that a doctor, nurse or health visitor accompany the police officer who is executing the warrant (if that officer so chooses) to gain entry into premises or access to the child. In fact the guidance recommends that such a direction be included as a matter of good practice (Vol. I, para. 4.56 and Section 48(11)).

Court directions: medical and psychiatric examinations and assessments

To ensure that children are not subjected to repeated and intrusive examinations the court has wide powers to give such directions (if any) as it considers appropriate with respect to the medical, psychiatric examination or other assessment of the child. These can be given either when the order is made, or subsequently, and can be varied at any time. They can also be very detailed and could, for example, prohibit any type of examination or assessment or direct that they should only take place with the court's permission. Alternatively the court may direct that the child's GP observe or participate in the examination. Note that the guidance recommends that directions be given whenever such examinations are likely to be an issue (Vol. 1, para. 4.63).

Although consent to the examinations or assessment can be given by the applicant as they have acquired parental responsibility, directions do not override the right of mature 'Gillick competent' under-16-year-olds and competent young people over 16 to refuse to submit to them.

Directions can also be given as to the contact which is, or is not, to be allowed between the child and any named person. Subject to this the Act requires reasonable contact to be maintained between the child and a range of people, including his or her parents, those with parental responsibility and any person with whom the child was living immediately before the order was made.

Discharge of an emergency protection order

There is no right of appeal against the making, or refusal to make, an EPO. However, an application can be made for it to be discharged by a wide range of people, such as the child, his or her parents, those with parental responsibility or anyone with whom the child was living before the order was made, except where the person making the application was given notice of and attended court when the order was made. Furthermore, no discharge application can be heard until 72 hours after the order was made.

Action after an emergency protection order

An EPO must be followed by investigations (*see* Section 47, Chapter 7). This may identify a need for further compulsory measures, such as interim care or supervision. Alternatively it may result in the child returning home without the need for any further intervention. In some cases voluntary services may be provided under Part III of the Act (*see* Chapter 5).

PRACTICE NOTES

Health professionals are likely to have a key role to play in the following aspects of an EPO.

Investigation: prior to the application. An application for an EPO by a local authority should always be preceded by an investigation under Section 47. Health professionals may thus be required to co-operate and collaborate with the local authority in the investigative process, particularly in:

- exchanging information
- checking records
- contributing to the child protection conference (and any review)
- being interviewed.

Grounds for an order. Professional expertise may be required in advising whether the grounds for an order have been met, both in 'frustrated access' cases where very fine judgements may need to be made as to whether an EPO or CAO is more appropriate, and in predicting whether significant harm is likely.

Court directions: medical and psychiatric examinations and assessments. The court may need to take professional advice about the nature, scope and objective of examinations and assessments and the detailed directions the order should contain.

Before examining or assessing a child, health professionals should ascertain:

- who has parental responsibility
- who has the right to consent (court directions do not override the rights of mature children to refuse to submit to examinations or assessments)
- whether specific directions have been given
- whether the examination or assessment is to be used in court proceedings.

When carrying out the examination or assessment health professionals should comply with any specified directions and consider whether they should be varied.

Police powers

The police may not only be involved in enforcing and applying for emergency protection orders but can also, as under the previous law, initiate their own protective action. Section 46 of the Act gives them the right to remove children to suitable alternative accommodation, keep them away from home and prevent them from leaving hospital or another place whenever they believe that the child would otherwise be likely to suffer significant harm.

The police do not need the court's permission to exercise these powers but such 'police protection' is only intended to be a very short-term measure. It cannot last more than 72 hours and does not involve any transfer of parental responsibility, although it does permit the 'designated officer' to do what is necessary for the child's welfare.

Under the Police and Criminal Evidence Act 1984 (Section 17) the police may enter and search premises without a warrant in order to save 'life and limb'. This is a particularly useful power if they need to gain access to a child before taking him or her into police protection.

Whilst the police are exercising their protective powers a number of duties must be undertaken. These are set out in detail in the Act and include informing the local authority of the steps taken, giving details of the child's accommodation, making enquiries, notifying the child's parents or those with parental responsibility and anyone with whom the child was living, and ascertaining the child's wishes and feelings.

Once enquiries have been completed by the designated officer the child should be released unless the child is still likely to suffer significant harm. If so, an application can be made for an EPO on behalf of the local authority.

The Act also deals with contact arrangements during police protection. There is a positive duty to allow the child contact with a wide range of people, including his or her parents, and those with parental responsibility, providing such contact is in the child's best interests.

PRACTICE NOTES

Health professionals may be required to examine, assess or treat a child in police protection. Before undertaking any such procedures they should ascertain:

- who has parental responsibility
- who has the right to consent.

Recovery of abducted, missing or runaway children

The Act contains three provisions designed to protect abducted, missing or runaway children. Although these generally re-enact existing law some important changes have been introduced. The most significant of these is the long-awaited provision regulating 'safe houses'.

Abduction

Section 49 makes it an offence to abduct a child or induce, assist or incite him or her to run away. The offence is only committed if done 'knowingly and without lawful authority or reasonable excuse'.

Recovery order

Section 50 enables the court to make a recovery order in respect of children in care, police protection or subject to an emergency protection order who have been abducted, have run away or are missing. The order's main effect is to authorize the removal of a child and to require disclosure of his or her whereabouts. In addition it gives the police powers of entry and search.

Children's refuges

Section 51 covers so-called 'safe houses' for runaway children. It enables such accommodation, which may include a foster home, to be given a certificate. The effect is to exempt those running the home from prosecution from various offences such as abduction. Strict regulations govern the running of these refuges (The Refuges (Children's Homes and Foster Placements) Regulations 1991) which are only intended to provide short-term help to those who otherwise would be at 'risk of harm'.

PRACTICE NOTES

Health professionals may be called upon to provide medical assistance to 'recovered' children and those in refuges. Before undertaking any examination, assessment or treatment they should ascertain:

- who has parental responsibility
- who has the right to consent.

Case studies

Case study 14

Patrick is just over two years old. His mother, Rosy, is 19 and four months pregnant. Rosy lives in a tower-block and is finding it very difficult to cope despite lots of support from social services. Patrick's father left over a year ago and Rosy has not seen him since then. A couple of months ago she kicked out her boyfriend when she discovered that he had been stealing from her purse and spending the money on drink. She does not expect to see him again.

Patrick is a sickly child, with constant chest infections. Tessa, the health visitor, and the practice nurse think he needs to be monitored very carefully as they suspect he may be failing to thrive. Patrick's GP is not convinced of this but agrees Patrick needs to have a full assessment as soon as possible.

Tessa discusses her concerns with Rosy and makes arrangements for Patrick to come to the surgery. Rosy fails to turn up. Several other appointments are made, all of which Rosy fails to keep either because Patrick was asleep and she did not want to disturb him or because she got the times muddled up. Finally she promises that she will definitely take him to the surgery the next day and Tessa arranges to pick her up at home. But when she gets there Rosy says she cannot come in as the flat is in a dreadful state. Tessa is becoming increasingly anxious about Patrick.

1. Tessa is uncertain about reporting her suspicions, especially as the GP is much less concerned about Patrick. What should she do?
2. Does Tessa have a duty to investigate Patrick's circumstances?
3. Does Tessa have a right to enter Rosy's home?
4. If Rosy again fails to keep her appointment what action should be taken?
5. What action should be taken if Rosy refuses to open the door to Tessa and a neighbour tells her that she has heard some very loud bangs and that Patrick has been screaming all night?
6. Does an emergency protection order give Tessa the right to enter Rosy's home without her authority?
7. If a warrant for police assistance is obtained to enforce the emergency protection order can it include a direction that Tessa should accompany the police?

Solutions

1. Tessa should refer her concerns to one or more of the agencies with statutory duties and/or powers to investigate and intervene, ie social services, NSPCC or the police, in accordance with locally agreed procedures.

    Following referral she should contribute to the enquiries and investigations which the local authority has a duty to make in order to decide what action it should take to promote or safeguard Patrick's welfare.

2. Local authorities have the primary responsibility for child protection but the Children Act expects other agencies to co-operate. This is why Section 47 enables local authorities to call upon health authorities, amongst others, 'to assist them with their enquiries (in particular by providing relevant information and advice)'.

3. Tessa has no right to enter Rosy's home – to do so an emergency protection order should be sought.

4. If access to Patrick is not an emergency because there are no urgent fears for his safety but it seems clear that attempts to arrange a voluntary assessment have failed, a child assessment order should be sought. Tessa cannot apply for a child assessment order herself as it can only be granted to a local authority or NSPCC.

5. In these circumstances, where there are urgent fears for Patrick's welfare, an emergency protection order should be sought. Tessa can apply for one herself 'if there is reasonable cause to believe that Patrick is likely to suffer significant harm if he is not removed'. But in the vast majority of cases the applicant will either be the local authority or the NSPCC.

    However, Tessa cannot apply for an emergency protection order just because she cannot see Patrick, only the local authority or NSPCC can apply for one in these kinds of circumstances.

6. An emergency protection order does not automatically authorize entry into Rosy's home without permission. If entry is likely to be refused the force of an order should be strengthened by permitting the applicant to enter premises and search for the child and/or by attaching a warrant for police assistance. In addition, the police have a right to enter premises without a warrant to save life or limb under the Police and Criminal Evidence Act 1984 which is unaffected by the Children Act.

7. Yes, this kind of direction can be included. Alternatively the warrant could direct that a GP or nurse accompany the police.

Case study 15

Roma is four years old and Sam is nearly two. Their mother, Thelma, lives with her boyfriend, Uriah, who is Sam's but not Roma's father. One morning Thelma turns up at the surgery in a terrible state. She has a black eye, a front tooth missing and cuts and bruises all over her arms. Roma also seems to be in a serious state. She is very pale and withdrawn, refuses to talk to Vera, the practice nurse whom she knows very well, and has a very large bruise on her forehead. She is also limping badly and has what seems to be several small now healing burns on her hands. Sam is playing happily and appears to be in fine shape.

Vera and the GP think that Thelma should go to hospital immediately with Roma but Winifred, the health visitor, wants to examine Roma and Sam first. When she suggests this Thelma starts crying and says 'He'll murder me if I go to hospital, I've got to get home quickly before he comes home for lunch'. She then grabs the children and starts to leave.

1. Can Winifred examine Roma and Sam without Thelma's consent?
2. Can Vera or the GP force Thelma to take Roma to casualty? If not, can either of them take her there instead?
3. If Uriah turns up and insists on taking Roma and Sam home, can he?
4. Is there any action that can be taken to stop Thelma taking Roma home (or to remove her once she returned home)?
5. What action should be taken in respect of Sam?

Solutions

1. Winifred has no right to examine either Roma or Sam without the consent of someone with parental responsibility (ie Thelma in respect of both Roma and Sam since it is assumed that in neither case has their father acquired parental responsibility). Without the necessary consent an emergency protection order or child assessment order would have to be obtained.
2. Neither Vera nor the GP can legally insist that Thelma takes Roma to hospital. Nor do they have the right to take her there themselves. Again they would have to obtain a court order, ie an emergency protection order.
3. Uriah is not Roma's father so unless he has acquired parental responsibility for her, for example, through a residence order, he has no authority to take her home without Thelma's permission. Even though Uriah is Sam's father he does not automatically have parental responsibility for him. So again, unless he has acquired it in some way (eg because he made a parental responsibility agreement with Thelma) he has no right to remove Sam without Thelma's consent.
4. An emergency protection order could be sought to stop Roma being removed if the situation was considered an emergency. An emergency protection order can be used either to keep a child in a safe place or to remove her to one. Similarly, if urgent action was needed when Roma returned home, an emergency protection order could be used to remove her. The police could also use their powers to remove or keep Roma safe if they had 'resonable cause to believe that she would otherwise be likely to suffer significant harm'.
5. Sam seems to be in less immediate danger than Roma but it may well be advisable to give him a full assessment as soon as possible. Efforts should be made to persuade Thelma to co-operate and bring Sam for an assessment. If she refuses and Vera, the GP or Winifred think that a full examination is necessary the criteria for a child assessment order may be fulfilled.

Case study 16(a)

Tracy is eight years old. She lives with her parents, a young married couple who have a very stormy relationship. Over the last few weeks Tracy's teacher has become increasingly concerned about her behaviour and suspects that she may have been sexually abused by her father. She discusses her suspicions with the school nurse who agrees that there is cause for concern. They decide to refer the case to the local authority.

Investigations result in the local authority obtaining an emergency protection order and Verona, a GP, is authorized by the order to go with social workers when it is exercised. On arrival at Tracy's flat, her parents let the social workers and GP in but refuse to let Verona examine Tracy.

1. Who has parental responsibility under the emergency protection order?
2. What medical procedures can be undertaken at this stage by Verona?
3. What is the effect of Tracy's parents refusing to allow Tracy to be examined?
4. What difference would it make if Tracy was aged 13 and refused to be examined?
5. If Tracy was 13 and court directions authorizing medical tests had been included in a child assessment order, would she have the right to refuse to submit to them?

Solutions

1. An emergency protection order gives parental responsibility to the local authority but it is limited to what 'is reasonably required to safeguard or promote' Tracy's welfare.

    Tracy's parents would retain their parental responsibility but their ability to exercise it would be very limited. For example, if Tracy was removed from home they would not be able to care for her and their contact with her might also be restricted.
2. Although the local authority's parental responsibility would allow it to authorize examinations to obtain evidence for court proceedings, the court's leave is required if the results are to be admissible. However, in all cases where such examinations are likely to be an issue, directions regulating medical or psychiatric examinations or other assessments are likely to be included in the emergency protection order itself. If so, they must be complied with or subsequently varied in ways permitted by the Children Act.
3. Since an emergency protection order gives limited parental responsibility to the local authority, including the right to consent to medical tests (*see* 2 above), Tracy's parent's objections can be overridden.
4. The Act clearly states that a child of sufficient understanding to make an informed decision can refuse to submit to any medical, psychiatric examination or assessment ordered by the court in an emergency protection order. Whether Tracy at 13 has reached the required level of understanding is a matter for the health professionals carrying out the examinations to decide. If she has, her refusal should be reported back to the court.

5. As with an emergency protection order, the Act clearly states that a child with sufficient understanding to make an informed decision can refuse to submit to any examinations directed in a child assessment order. Therefore, if Tracy is considered sufficiently mature to refuse, her wishes must be respected.

Case study 16(b)

Tracy's injuries were worse than expected and it is necessary to keep her in hospital for a few days. Whilst there it soon becomes clear to Winston, the consultant paediatrician, that the emergency order needs to be extended, primarily so that further examinations can be carried out. There is also a problem with visits as Tracy's father turns up at very inconvenient times and demands to see Tracy immediately, claiming that he has the right to see his daughter whenever he likes. Tracy tells a nurse, Una, that she does not want to see her father for at least a few days.

1. How long does an emergency protection order initially last? Can it be extended?
2. When can an application be made to court to vary medical directions? Can Winston make the application?
3. What contact rights do Tracy's parents have whilst the emergency protection order is in force? Will hospital staff be involved in deciding what contact arrangements are best?
4. What action should be taken when the emergency protection order expires?

Solutions

1. An emergency protection order lasts initially for eight days, although a shorter period can be specified in the order. It can be extended only once, for up to seven days.
2. If it seems that the original medical directions are not appropriate, an application can be made to vary them at any time whilst the order remains in force. Those entitled to seek a variation include a variety of people such as the parties to the proceedings and the local authority. Any person named in the direction, such as Winston if so-named, or any other expert directed to carry out the assessment would also be able to apply for a variation.
3. Whilst an emergency protection order lasts parents, amongst others, are entitled to 'reasonable' contact with their child unless it has been curtailed or otherwise restricted by court directions. What is reasonable depends upon the circumstances of the case. As Tracy seems reluctant to see her father it may be appropriate to only allow telephone contact. Note also, that if contact is likely to be problematic it is advisable to seek court directions so that priorities for contact can be established and specifically included in the order – they can always be varied if necessary. Hospital staff, especially Una, may be asked to advise on the effect of current contact arrangements and what changes should be made.

4. Action after the expiry of an emergency protection order depends on the results of the various medical tests and on whether voluntary support is considered adequate. Alternatively an interim care order may be appropriate. In any event the Act requires local authorities to make further enquiries after they have obtained an emergency protection order.

9

Children Looked After
by Local Authorities

When children are being 'looked after' by a local authority, a series of provisions come into operation which specify how they should be treated. Although most of these provisions existed in previous legislation some important reforms have been introduced. The most significant features of the new statutory framework are as follows.

1. Change of terminology

The phrase 'looked after' is a new term which is intended to cover two main groups of children: those accommodated by voluntary arrangement and those in care as a result of a care order. Other children who are kept away from home such as those on remand, in police protection or subject to an emergency protection order are also included in the definition.

2. Change of emphasis

More emphasis is now placed on the need to make detailed written plans for children in partnership with them, their parents, and other people who are important to them. This means consulting and notifying them about decisions, encouraging and maintaining family links and working towards the family's eventual reunification. It also means giving parents and children greater opportunities to question local authority decision-making, hence the new requirement to set up formal complaint procedures. The duties of local authorities to prepare children for leaving care and to provide them with after-care services have also been strengthened.

3. Comprehensive responsibilities

Although the Act distinguishes more clearly between children voluntarily accommodated and those in care as a result of a court order, the responsibilities owed to both sets of children are in many respects the same. However, local authorities do have some additional duties and powers in relation to children in care because a care order gives them parental responsibility. Overall, the intention behind the reformed scheme is to ensure that the needs of all children are met, regardless of how they came to be looked after and to provide a coherent statutory framework within which the local authority can work and act as 'good parents'.

Most of the law governing how children should be cared for is contained in Part III of the Act (Sections 22–26) and Schedule 2, Part II and III. Various sets of regulations also apply, likewise guidance volumes 3 and 4. Other related guidance documents are *The care of children, principles and practice in regulations and guidance*, HMSO, 1990 and *Patterns and outcomes in child placement*, HMSO, 1991.

This chapter will consider the local authority's responsibilities under four broad headings: general welfare; contact; accommodation; and planning.

General welfare (Section 22)

In summary local authorities must:

- safeguard and promote the welfare of each child
- make such use of services available for children cared for by their own parents as appears reasonable
- consult the child, his or her parents, those with parental responsibility and others 'considered relevant' before making any decision with respect to the child
- give due consideration to the wishes and feelings of the child and other persons consulted in making any such decision
- give due consideration to the child's religious persuasion, racial origin and cultural and linguistic background
- prepare all children they look after for leaving care and provide them and certain other young people, with after-care services
- establish a formal procedure for dealing with complaints and representations.

Note that these general welfare duties are also owed by voluntary organizations and registered children homes.

'Contact' and related duties (Schedule 2, Part II)

Local authorities must:

- endeavour to promote contact between the child and his or her parents, those with parental responsibility and any relative, friend or other person connected with him or her, unless it is not reasonably practicable or consistent with his or her welfare
- take such steps as are reasonably practicable to ensure the child's parents and those with parental responsibility are kept informed of where he or she is being accommodated (note that this duty does not apply if the child is in care and it is felt that such information would prejudice the child's welfare)

- appoint an independent visitor where it appears:
  - i that communication between a child and a parent or person with parental responsibility has been infrequent or
  - ii that he or she has not visited, been visited by, or lived with any such person during the preceding 12 months.

Other related contact provisions include the duty to promote contact whilst a child is in care (*see* Section 34 and Chapter 7) and the requirement to consider contact arrangements when making plans for the child (*see* below).

Accommodation and placement duties (Section 23)

Local authorities must:

- provide accommodation (local authorities can discharge this duty in a number of ways, *see* Chapter 10)
- maintain children (apart from providing accommodation)
- give priority to placements with, amongst others, a parent, non-parent with parental responsibility, relative, or other person connected with the child, unless that would not be reasonably practicable or consistent with his or her welfare
- ensure that children are accommodated near their home and that siblings are accommodated together
- ensure that accommodation for disabled children is not unsuitable for their particular needs.

PRACTICE NOTES

Health professionals may be asked to co-operate with local authorities in carrying out any of their responsibilities towards children they look after, particularly in relation to the following:

- ensuring that communication and consultation with parents and children is effective – professional expertise may, for example, be essential if a child has communication difficulties or complex needs
- advising on proposed contact arrangements and/or whether existing arrangements are working satisfactorily
- preparing children for leaving care and providing after-care support, notably on health and related matters
- helping to formulate complaints which may arise on health care issues
- advising on the suitability of placements and whether existing arrangements should be changed.

Planning duties

The Act now requires 'responsible authorities' (local authorities, voluntary organizations and registered children's homes) to make immediate and long-term arrangements for a child's care. In particular they must draw up an individual plan in writing for each child whom they are proposing to look after. The purpose of the plan is 'to help focus work with the family and child and prevent drift'. 'Drift' is a word coined in the 1970s to highlight the plight of children who spent most of their childhood in care, not as a result of a decision that this would be the best outcome, but by default.

The new emphasis on planning is also intended to ensure that children and their parents are more involved in decision-making. As the guidance states

> 'planning with the involvement of parents will provide the basis of partnership between the responsible authorities and parents and child and should enable the placement to proceed positively' (Vol. 3, para. 2.11).

Accordingly, regulations stipulate that when children are voluntarily accommodated arrangements for their care must be agreed, as far as is reasonably practicable, with them (if they are over 16) and with any person with parental responsibility or their carers. However, where a child is looked after under a care order there is no obligation to agree a plan, although the guidance recommends that such agreement should be sought as a matter of good practice.

Contents of the plan

Although there is no prescribed format for the plan, the Arrangements for the Placement of Children (General) Regulations 1991 specify the matters to be covered. These include educational and health care considerations and requirements (*see* below), arrangements for contact and immediate and long-term objectives. Unsurprisingly, distinctions are made between children subject to a court order and those provided with accommodation voluntarily. For example, the plan for the latter must contain details of – amongst other things – the respective responsibilities of the authority, child and parents, contact arrangements and the expected duration of the placement.

Health considerations (Regulation 4 and Schedule 2)

When making a plan for a child, responsible authorities must consider:

- the child's state of health
- the child's health history
- the effect of the child's health and health history on his or her development
- existing arrangements for the child's medical and dental care, treatment and surveillance
- the possible need for appropriate action which should be identified to assist necessary change of such care, treatment or surveillance

- the possible need for preventive measures such as vaccination and immunization, and screening for vision and hearing.

Health requirements (Regulation 7)

This regulation imposes two quite specific duties, both of which must be carried out as far as reasonably practicable before a placement and if that is not possible as soon as reasonably practicable thereafter. Responsible authorities must:

- ensure that arrangements are made for the child to be medically examined
- ensure that a written assessment of the child's state of health and need for health care is provided by the practitioner who carried out the examination unless this has been done within the previous three months or the child refuses consent (assuming he or she is mature enough to make that decision).

In addition, the above regulation also states that children must be provided with health care services, including medical and dental care and treatment, during the placement.

Notification (Regulation 5)

Responsible authorities must notify the district health authority and the child's GP, among others, in writing of the contents of the plan preferably before the placement is made.

Detailed guidance on how these health care regulations should actually be applied are contained in Vol. 3, paras. 2.23–32. The following is a summary.

PRACTICE NOTES

'Arrangements for ensuring that children receive proper health care during placement will involve the responsible authority, parents, the child, other carer, GP, community child health doctor, health visitor, the school health service and, depending on the child's needs, specialist and domiciliary services'.

In particular it means that

- a 'positive approach' to the child's health should be adopted to include general surveillance and care for health and developmental progress as well as treatment for illness and accidents
- the child should be registered with a GP and a contract entered into with a general dental practitioner
- NHS provision and school health services should be used in the same way as for any other child
- an especially 'informed and sensitive' approach should be adopted since children who are looked after 'will often have suffered early disadvantage and may be at risk because they have not received continuity of care'

- any special health care needs of children from ethnic minority groups should be met, if necessary by putting carers in touch with a named health professional
- responsible authorities and health authorities should aim to develop effective arrangements for the communication of information relating to the child's health to (and between) all the health professionals who are involved with the child
- policies and procedures on consent to examination and treatment should be clear and made known to the health authority, the child's carers and relevant health professionals
- arrangements should be set out clearly in each plan or agreement and should enable appropriate health care to be obtained 'without confusion or delay'
- the need for operations and major treatment should be discussed with parents and their consent obtained, subject to the exercise of local authorities' overriding powers in respect of children in care and the rights of mature young people (ie those over 16 and under 16 if 'Gillick competent') to refuse consent.

Reviewing the plan

Regular, structured and comprehensive reviews of children's care have long been recognized as the only effective way to monitor their progress, make informed decisions in the light of changed circumstances and prevent 'drift'. Under previous legislation, however, review obligations were often ignored, largely because there was little guidance on how they should be carried out and what they should cover. Accordingly the Act introduces much more stringent requirements about reviews, which are now governed by the Review of Children's Cases Regulations 1991, and associated guidance (Vols. 3 and 4). The regulations specify, amongst other things, the frequency and form of reviews, and what matters should be considered (ie education, contact and health arrangements, who should be consulted and who should attend review meetings).

Health considerations (Regulation 5)

When reviewing a case responsible authorities must consider the same health care matters as in the planning regulations (*see* above, Regulation 4 and Schedule 2).

Health reviews (Regulation 6)

During a placement responsible authorities must ensure that children under two years old are medically examined every six months and that a written assessment is provided of their state of health and need for health care. For older children this must be done once a year, unless the child is of 'sufficient understanding' and refuses consent.

PRACTICE NOTES

Until the child is at school, medical examination and written health assessments should take place and use, wherever possible, any appropriate information gained from the schedule of development surveillance prescribed by the district health authority in which the child is placed. It is also recommended that medical examination and assessment should precede any change of school or at intervals specified in the child's plan (Vol. 4, para. 2.28).

Health professionals may also be asked to:

- carry out required examinations and submit written assessments
- exchange information
- interpret health reports and information
- assist in decision-making, for example, by participating and contributing to the review meeting.

Before carrying out any required examinations health professionals should establish who has parental responsibility and the right to consent.

Case studies

Case study 17

Victoria is 12 years old. She has just been made the subject of a care order because of sexual abuse by her stepfather. The abuse only came to light when she was admitted to hospital after falling off her bicycle. Victoria has been traumatized by her experiences but fortunately she seems to be settling in well with her new foster parents. Her GP, Wendy, however, thinks that she needs to be medically examined as soon as possible. Victoria refuses.

1. Can Wendy insist that Victoria is examined?
2. Who has the right to consent to such an examination?
3. Would it make any difference if a care order had not been made but instead Victoria was being voluntarily accommodated?
4. What if Victoria was only five years old but still refused to be examined?
5. What action should be taken if Victoria does agree to be examined but Wendy is unhappy about the health care arrangements which have been made for her?

Solutions

1. Once a care order is made in respect of Victoria the local authority must draw up an individual plan for her. Health considerations are an important part of the plan and regulations provide for children to be medically examined either before they are placed or as soon as possible thereafter.

    However, children need not be examined if they have been examined within the last three months and a written assessment has been made about their health. Nor is placement prohibited if it is impossible to persuade Victoria to be examined.

2. Regulations clearly state that children of sufficient understanding can refuse to be examined. This means that if Victoria is considered mature enough to make an

informed decision her wishes must be respected. But if Wendy does not think she is then consent would have to be obtained from someone with parental responsibility (the local authority).

3. If Victoria was being provided with accommodation under a voluntary arrangement the same health care provisions would apply and she should be medically examined, unless this has already been done within the last three months and a written assessment has been made. However, she would have the right to refuse such examinations providing she was considered mature enough.

4. If Victoria was only five years old and subject to a care order then consent for the examination would have to be obtained from anyone with parental responsibility (the local authority). If she was being voluntarily accommodated consent could not be obtained from the local authority since it would not have parental responsibility, but it could be obtained from someone with parental responsibility such as her mother. If she refused, appropriate court orders could be applied for (eg a child assessment order).

5. If Wendy's concerns cannot be resolved satisfactorily she could consider making a complaint under the local authority's complaint procedure.

Case study 18

William is 17 years old. For the last four months he has been accommodated by X Health Authority. He has recently moved out of their care and has asked the local authority for after-care advice and assistance. The local authority has very limited funds to resource such provision and William is told that they are under no obligation to provide such services.

Are they obliged? Would it make any difference if William had previously been accommodated by the local authority or by, or on behalf of, a voluntary organization?

Solutions

Complex provisions contained in Section 24 of the Children Act govern after-care provision. Basically local authorities must 'advise and befriend' young people under 21 who, at any time between the ages of 16 and 18, were looked after by a local authority or by, or on behalf of, a voluntary organization, but only when the following conditions are satisfied:

*   if the local authority knows they are in the area
*   they have asked for help
*   they appear to need advice and befriending
*   (where relevant) those who were looking after them do not have the facilities to provide after-care.

In addition, local authorities can – but are not obliged – to offer similar services to a group of other young people who fulfil the same conditions but who were cared for in other establishments, notably, registered children's homes, private foster homes or, for a consecutive period of at least three months, by any health or education authority or in any residential care home, nursing home or mental nursing home.

In applying these provisions to William, provided he satisfies the specified conditions, we see that he may be provided with after-care services if accommodated by X Health Authority, and must be so provided if he has been accommodated by the local authority or a voluntary organization.

10

The Legal Regulation of
Substitute Care

A substantial part of the Children Act deals with the legal regulation of the various different forms of substitute care which can be provided for children living or cared for outside the family home. Although most of the law considered in this chapter consolidates and re-enacts previous legislation some important reforms have been introduced, notably in relation to child-minding and children's homes. Overall these aim to strengthen and widen the regulatory framework and to ensure that uniform standards apply to all facilities. The various different forms of care are as follows.

Children's homes

There are three categories of children's homes:

- community homes – provided either by local authorities or voluntary organizations
- voluntary homes – provided by non-profit making voluntary organizations such as Barnado's
- registered children's homes – private homes run for profit which accommodate more than three children at any one time (this category also includes small independent boarding schools with between four and 50 boarders).

Although the great majority (80%) of children are in community homes of various kinds, the Act attempts to ensure parity of treatment for all children looked after in residential accommodation. Accordingly it provides that:

1. Except for the duty to provide after-care services, voluntary organizations (Section 61) and persons running registered children's homes (Section 64) owe children the same broad and general welfare duties as local authorities (*see* Chapter 9).

2. All children's homes are governed by the Arrangements for the Placement of Children (General) Regulations 1991 and the Review of Children's Cases Regulations 1991. This means that individual written plans must be made for each child and regularly reviewed (*see* Chapter 9).

3. Complaints procedures must be set up in all children's homes.

4. All children's homes are governed by the Children's Homes Regulations 1991 (*see* below).

Role of local authorities

Local authorities have substantial supervisory powers over children's homes. Registration, as before, is the key regulatory mechanism which applies to both private and voluntary homes. In addition local authorities must ensure that the welfare of the children accommodated is being safeguarded and promoted. Regular visiting is also obligatory, backed up by entry and inspection powers.

PRACTICE NOTES

Medical assistance. Doctors, nurses and health visitors may be directed (by a court) to accompany the police when a warrant for police assistance is exercised. A warrant may be necessary when a children's home is being inspected but entry to the premises, or access to the children, is refused or seems likely to be refused.

Conduct and administration of children's homes

Children's homes are described in the guidance as a 'vital resource' and a 'positive and desirable way of providing stability and care' which should not only 'set out to treat each child as an individual person but also exercise the concern that a good parent would by providing a safe environment which promotes the child's development and protects him from exposure to harm in his contacts with other people or experiences in the community'.

To ensure that children's homes achieve these broad aims the Act establishes a new statutory framework. This consists of a new set of regulations: The Children's Homes Regulations 1991 and detailed guidance (Vol. 4). Further proposals are contained in the *Utting Report: children in the public care*, 1991.

The regulations deal with such matters as staffing, standard of accommodation, control and discipline, employment and education, religious observance, food provision, purchase of clothes, record keeping, procedures to be followed if a child absconds, visiting, inspection and registration. There are also various health-related regulations.

Control and discipline (Regulation 8)

This regulation prohibits any form of corporal punishment and various other specified measures such as intimate physical searches or examinations or the use, or the withholding of, medication or medical and dental treatment. Such actions are described as 'dangerous and utterly unacceptable practices totally forbidden in all circumstances, whether as a disciplinary measure or otherwise to control the child' (Vol. 4, para. 1.91). Even so, these measures can be used by, or in accordance with, the instructions of a doctor or dentist – but only when it is necessary to protect the child's health or where immediate action is necessary to prevent harm to any person or serious damage to property. If sanctions are administered a record must be kept, which should include the child's name, details of the inappropriate behaviour, names of staff present, and date and nature of the sanction.

Storage of medicinal products (Regulation 9)

This regulation specifies that medicinal products must be stored in a secure place so as to prevent children having access to them unless under the supervision of a member of staff. In addition they must only be administered by a member of staff, nurse or doctor, unless:

- they are stored (by the child for whom they are provided) in such a way that others are prevented from using them, and
- they can be safely self-administered by that child.

The guidance recommends that young people over 16 should in general be entrusted with the retention and administration of their own medication and be provided with a secure place to keep it where necessary. Each home should also lay down procedures for the administration of medications and keep records of all medicine given, including the date and circumstances of its administration and by whom it was administered. Details of self-administered medicine should also be recorded (Regulation 17 and Schedule 3).

Confidential records (health aspects, Regulation 15 and Schedule 2)

This regulation requires an individual confidential case record to be kept for each child for 75 years. The following health-related details must be included:

- any special dietary or health needs of the child
- details of any immunization, illness, allergy, or medical examination of the child and of any medical or dental need of the child
- details of any health examination or developmental test conducted with respect to the child at or in connection with his or her school
- the name and address of the doctor with whom the child is registered
- details of all medicinal products taken by the child while in the home and by whom they were administered, including those which the child was permitted to self-administer him or herself
- details of any accident involving the child.

According to the guidance (Vol. 4, para. 1.99) health records should build on earlier records. If these are not available efforts should be made to obtain them. They should also be regularly updated with all relevant information about health needs and development, illnesses, operations, immunizations, allergies, medications and dates of appointments with GPs and specialists. The records should not, however, record the antibody status of a child who is HIV positive as this information should be held on a need-to-know basis only. Furthermore, authorities are expected to ensure that staff are aware of issues surrounding HIV and AIDS and take appropriate precautions in all cases to avoid situations which could result in the transmission of HIV infection. When the child leaves the home the records should be made available to whoever is to have subsequent care of the child.

Notification of significant events (Regulation 19)

This regulation requires certain specified 'significant' events affecting children living in a home to be notified to various people, including the district health authority within whose district the children's home is situated. These events are the death of a child or serious harm to a child, any serious accident, any serious illness, and the outbreak in the home of any notifiable infectious disease to which the Public Health (Control of Disease) Act 1984 applies or disease to which provisions of that Act are applied by the Public Health (Infectious Disease) Regulations 1988 (5.1 1988/1546).

PRACTICE NOTES

Health professionals may be involved in various aspects of these health-related regulations, especially if it is thought appropriate to use (or withhold) medication or treatment. The compilation of accurate health records may also require their assistance.

Note also that the health-related aspects of the planning and review regulations which apply to children's homes have implications for professional practice. In particular these require, for example, regular medical examinations and written reports (see Chapter 9).

Other implications for health professionals arise from the additional health care guidance given (Vol. 4, para. 1.92 – 104) to compensate for the 'poverty of expectation' about the standard of health children in homes should enjoy and because they may be 'particularly vulnerable' due to lack of continuity of health care. The following recommendations are made:

1. *Adoption of a proactive approach on health issues.* This means promoting all aspects of children's health with the 'same assiduity as would be the case for children living with caring parents'. Health professionals may be asked, for example, to advise on alcohol and other substance abuse, sexual matters, and HIV/AIDS as well as treatment of illness and accidents.

2. *Vigilant attitudes.* To remedy deficiencies in past medical care, careful and continuous monitoring of children's health is urged as is seeking prompt medical advice when causes of concern are identified.

3. *Co-operation and effective communication.* Close collaboration and co-operation is necessary between those with parental responsibility, the staff in the home, and relevant health professionals, especially when children have special health care needs such as diabetes, epilepsy or haemophilia, thalassaemia and sickle cell anaemia.

Accommodation provided by a health authority

Section 85 contains important new provisions covering children accommodated by health authorities and NHS trusts (likewise education authorities) which bring such establishments within the protection of mainstream child care legislation for the first time. The reforms have three broad aims: to ensure that such children are not 'forgotten' and left to drift in institutional care (a not uncommon risk in the past when children were placed away from their homes in remote and rural areas); to encourage more coherent planning; and to enable local authorities to assess the quality of care provided. The new responsibilities are as follows.

Notification duty

Health and education authorities (including NHS trusts) must notify the responsible authority of children they have accommodated for a consecutive period of more than three months (school holidays do not count towards this period). The 'responsible authority' is the local authority for the area in which a child lives or was ordinarily resident immediately before being accommodated, or the one in whose area the accommodation is situated. They must also notify the responsible authority when such children cease to be accommodated.

Note also, the other notification duty imposed on health authorities, NHS trusts and LEAs (by Section 24 (12)) which requires them to inform the local authority when a young person of 16 leaves their accommodation (which has been provided for a consecutive three month period).

Role of local authorities

Once they have been notified, responsible authorities have two obligations:

- to take such steps as are reasonably practicable to enable them to determine whether the child's welfare is being adequately safeguarded and promoted
- to consider the extent to which, if at all, they should exercise any of their functions under the Act.

In addition, local authorities can provide after-care services for young people who leave health or education authority accommodation after the age of 16.

PRACTICE NOTES

Co-operation between authorities (including specialist advice through district handicap, child development and community mental handicap teams) is needed, especially where each agency is, or has been, actively involved with the child and his or her family. In particular the guidance recommends (Vol. 4, para. 1.195–205 and Vol. 6, para. 13.7–13) that local authorities:

- make enquiries (within 14 days of notification) in order to ascertain the circumstances of each child's case and assess what steps to take
- obtain written assurances from the health authority that proper parental contact and responsibility is established or is being maintained
- make suitable arrangements with health authorities to gain access to premises.

Co-operation between local authorities and health professionals is also urged to ensure that children receive the services they need and appropriate support when they return home, especially when their stay in hospital has been prolonged.

For further guidance see *The welfare of children and young people in hospital*, HMSO, 1991.

Residential care, nursing and mental nursing homes

In some cases children will need to live in one of these types of homes. Unless they are run by a local authority these homes must be registered and regulated under the Registered Homes Act 1984. To ensure that they are adequately cared for, however, the same notification duties are imposed (by Sections 86 and 24) on those running the homes as apply to those accommodated by health authorities (*see* above). Local authorities also have the same supervisory duties and powers to promote their welfare and provide after-care services. In addition they have a right of entry.

PRACTICE NOTES

Medical assistance. Doctors, nurses and health visitors may be directed by a court to accompany the police when a warrant for police assistance is exercised if entry is refused or is likely to be refused.

Independent schools

Independent schools with more than 50 boarders which are neither residential care homes nor children's homes are brought into the mainstream of the child care system for the first time by Section 87. This section imposes two new duties. The first requires school proprietors to promote and safeguard the welfare of the children they are accommodating. The second duty (which is essentially supervisory) requires local authorities to take reasonable steps to determine whether this duty is being complied with. They also have complementary powers of entry and inspection covering the premises, children and records.

Although there are no detailed regulations governing the management and conduct of independent schools, Volume 5 provides a basic framework of practice. Its main aim is to protect children from inappropriate care or abuse. It therefore covers such matters as standards of accommodation, staffing, health care (*see* below), contact with parents, personal relations and discipline, restriction of liberty, complaints procedure, religious and cultural ethos.

PRACTICE NOTES

Health care is dealt with in para. 3.5.1–5.7 and the following specific recommendations are made which may involve health professionals:

General health care:

- local authorities should report any health problems discovered during inspections to a school's proprietor and suggest that he or she refers the problem to the school medical officer, GP, school health service or environmental health department
- all children should normally be registered with a GP (usually, but not always, the school medical officer)
- the right of 16-year-olds and above to choose their own practitioner should be recognized
- schools should, if possible, have suitably qualified staff, such as nurses, to deal with health matters
- a system of notification should be set up to inform parents and guardians of deaths, accidents, serious illness, infectious diseases or other serious harm.

Health promotion:

- children should be actively encouraged to follow a healthy lifestyle with particular emphasis on a healthy diet, regular physical activity and the avoidance of smoking and excess alcohol
- an 'acceptable level' of hygiene should exist in all parts of the school
- the school medical officer should make regular inspections of food preparation areas, dining rooms, dormitories and washing facilities and advise the school accordingly.

Health facilities:
All but the smallest of schools are expected to have their own sanitoria, consulting room, treatment room and a secure, locked room or cupboard for medicines and drugs. If simple medication, such as paracetamol or cough linctus is administered by non-trained staff, then it too should be kept in a locked cupboard.

Child protection:
Schools are expected to have clearly laid down and recognized procedures for dealing with allegations of child abuse which should reflect those prescribed by the local Area

Child Protection Committee. Good practice within the school should provide for:

- a senior member of staff to be nominated for responsibility for child protection issues
- a detailed note to be made when abuse is alleged
- immediate notification to the local authority
- appropriate arrangements to be made for counselling the child and informing parents
- any complaint of abuse to be independently investigated (in accordance with ACPC procedures).

Inspection (physical examination):
Inspections are governed by regulations (Inspection of Premises, Children and Records (Independent Schools) Regulations 1991). These authorize inspection of records, premises and children. Note that the guidance states that where an inspection includes a physical examination this should be limited to a visual examination rather than a medical or intimate examination. Any examination is also subject to the child's consent where he or she is of sufficient understanding to give or withhold that consent. (*See* also *Inspecting independent schools with boarding: an induction framework for social services inspectors, trainers and managers*, DOH, 1992.)

Medical assistance:
Although there is no power for an authorized person (ie an inspector) to take a doctor with him or her, the guidance says that the local authority can designate a doctor as an authorized person instead of or in addition to a social worker.

In some cases, too, doctors, nurses or health visitors may be directed by a court to accompany the police when a warrant for police assistance is exercised in cases where entry to premises or access to children is refused or is likely to be refused.

Private fostering arrangements

Although parents cannot transfer or surrender their parental responsibility they can delegate it and arrange for someone else to exercise it on their behalf. When this involves full-time residential care arranged privately between individuals, it is called private fostering. Such arrangements are governed by Part IX and Schedules 7 and 8 of the Act and the Children (Private Arrangements for Fostering) Regulations 1991. Although these provisions largely repeat existing legislation some changes have been made. For example, the definition of a privately fostered child has been simplified. It now covers a child under 16 (or 18 if disabled) who is cared for by someone who is not a parent, relative (defined as a grandparent, brother, sister, uncle, aunt or step-parent) or non-parent with parental responsibility for at least 28 days.

Notification obligations requiring the local authority to be informed of placements remain, as before, the key regulatory control. They have, however, been broadened and apply to former and prospective foster parents and those with parental responsibility.

Role of local authorities

Local authorities are not responsible for selecting, registering or approving private foster parents but they do have an important supervisory function. The authorities have to satisfy themselves that the welfare of privately fostered children is being satisfactorily safeguarded and promoted and, they also have a new duty to make sure that necessary advice is given to all carers. Moreover they have the power to provide after-care services to privately fostered children.

Other responsibilities include regular visiting (regulations specify that if it is considered appropriate the child should be seen alone), report writing and powers of entry and inspection and so on. Local authorities can also invoke various mechanisms to control placements. Certain people are automatically disqualified from fostering, for example, unless they have obtained the local authority's prior consent. In addition, unsuitable placements can be prohibited or restricted, or specific requirements can be imposed. Note also, the provisions regulating fostering limits by which a person may not usually foster more than three children, although this can be exceeded in certain circumstances (*see* Schedule 7). Detailed guidance on all aspects of private fostering is contained in Volume 8.

PRACTICE NOTES

The guidance makes the following recommendations which may have implications for health professionals.

All agencies should liaise about the existence of private foster children of whom the social services may be unaware (Vol. 8, para. 1.6.21). A health professional may, for example, be the first to learn about privately fostered children. If so they should be alert to their needs and ensure that they do not miss out on health surveillance programmes.

Other more specific health-related regulations and recommendations which may involve health professionals are as follows.

Suitability of foster parents: Regulation 2 requires local authorities to assess the suitability of foster parents which involves making enquiries about, for example, parenting capacity, lifestyle and their ability to provide for the child's health care needs (medical examinations and assessments may be required as part of this process).

Health records and medical history: The guidance recommends that the personal child health record should be held by the foster parents and a full medical history of the child should be compiled. This should include not just basic details such as height and weight but also details of immunizations given and dates including, where practicable, the results of any neonatal screening tests; infectious diseases; in-patient or out-patient hospital treatment; congenital conditions which have or may have, medical implications and/or which necessitate ongoing health care; allergies (including allergies to medication); current short-term or long-term medication and other treatments (including consultants involved) and relevant information on any special dietary requirements or dietary restrictions.

Medical examination: Although medical examinations and reports are not legally required the guidance recommends that as a matter of 'good practice' children should be medically examined as soon as the fostering placement starts, or as soon as possible thereafter. Furthermore, where a child has an incomplete medical history local authorities should consider imposing a requirement (under Schedule 8) for further medical examination to be carried out at specified periods (Vol. 8, para. 1.7.12).

Consent to medical examination or treatment: General medical consent, in respect of treatment for which the child him or herself is not capable of giving consent, to cover everyday treatment which may become necessary should be given in writing to the foster parents. If appropriate, copies should be given to the health authority.

Registration with a GP: Regulation 2 requires a privately fostered child to be included on a GP's list, ideally his or her present one. Local authorities are expected to ensure in partnership with the family health services authority, that all children are so registered.

Female circumcision: Regulation 2 requires local authorities to satisfy themselves that a privately fostered child's needs arising from religious persuasion, racial origin and cultural and linguistic background are being met. This means:

- that health authorities should co-operate with local authorities in dealing with prohibited practices, such as female circumcision, and
- health professionals should be alert to the possibility of such practices.

Male circumcision: This is not prohibited but the guidance recommends that if a parent requests a foster parent to arrange it the circumcision should be carried out in an environment which provides adequate safeguards by a properly qualified medical practitioner at a hospital or clinic.

Health-related advice: Regulation 2 requires local authorities to satisfy themselves that private foster parents are being given necessary advice. Where appropriate this may include advice from health professionals, especially when a child has special needs or is 'in need' within the definition of the Act.

The guidance also recommends that all foster parents should have a working knowledge of, and skills in, first aid or be encouraged to obtain such knowledge.

Medical assistance: Doctors, nurses and health visitors may be directed by the court to accompany the police if a warrant for police assistance is granted to gain entry and carry out inspections.

Child-minding and day care

Part X and Schedule 9 contain important provisions designed to protect children who are looked after by child-minders or in day care facilities. Traditionally these forms of substitute care have been the least regulated and predictably the reforms introduced by the Act aim to strengthen controls and improve the regulatory and supervisory role of local authorities. In addition the new scheme should ensure that acceptable standards of care are set and complied with. Detailed guidance on standards is contained in Volume 2, Chapter 6 and registration and inspection requirements are covered in Volume 2, Chapters 7 and 8 and Volume 8, Chapter 3 (*see* also *Registration of childminding and day care*, DOH, 1991).

The basic regulatory mechanism is a modernized registration system under which local authorities have to keep an open register of child-minders and other providers of day care. They must also inspect all registered premises at least once a year (in addition to having other inspection powers) and can impose requirements to improve safety of premises or equipment, for example, as a condition of registration. Failure to register without reasonable excuse is a criminal offence.

For the purposes of the Act the following definitions apply:

- *Child-minder:* a person who looks after one or more children under the age of eight for reward for more than two hours a day in domestic premises (ie private accommodation). The definition excludes certain people, such as the child's parents, relatives and nannies.
- *Day care:* those who provide day care for children under the age of eight for more than two hours a day in non-domestic premises (for example, private nurseries and play groups). Again, a number of facilities are excluded from this definition including children's homes, health service hospitals, occasional crèches (*see* further Section 71 and Schedule 9).

PRACTICE NOTES

Health professionals may be involved in the following aspects:

Registration. Registration is governed by regulations which specify the information which must be provided about the applicant. This includes:

- *referees* – two names must be submitted (these may be health professionals)
- *GP* – the name and address of the applicant's GP must be provided but can only be contacted with the applicant's permission
- *health checks* – details about an applicant's health, covering serious illness over the previous five years, hospital admissions during the previous two years and any curent medical treatment, must be provided
- *cancellation or refusal of registration* – the views of health professionals may be sought in determining whether a child-minder or day-care provider (or their premises) are not up to the required standard.

Medical assistance. Doctors, nurses or health visitors may be directed by a court to accompany the police when a warrant for police assistance is granted to gain entry to premises in order to carry out inspections.

Foster placements

One of the ways in which local authorities can discharge their accommodation duties is to place children with 'local authority' foster parents. The Act defines such placements as those with a family, relative, friend or any other suitable person (unless he is a parent of the child, a person with parental responsibility for him or, where the child is in care, a person in whose favour there was a residence order in force immediately before the care order was made, Section 23).

Foster placements are a well-established part of child care practice and are increasingly popular. They account for nearly half of all children looked after by local authorities. They can be used for a wide variety of purposes, including short-term, temporary 'respite' or 'phased' care arrangements, or as long-term measures with a view to adoption.

Foster placements, whether made by a local authority or voluntary organizations, are governed by the Foster Placement (Children) Regulations 1991. These generally forbid placements with people who have not been approved and cover such matters as the selection, approval, supervision and termination of placements, record keeping, agreements, visiting requirements and so on. Fostering limits – usually three – are dealt with in Schedule 7.

There is also an important provision in Schedule 2(11) which requires local authorities – when making arrangements designed to encourage people to become foster parents – to have regard to the different racial groups to which the children in need within their area belong. Other guidance on foster placements is contained in Volume 3, Chapters 3 and 4. Finally it should be noted that individual written plans must be made for each fostered child and also be regularly reviewed. A complaints procedure must also be set up.

PRACTICE NOTES

The following aspects of the Foster Placement Regulations may have implications for health professionals.

Approval (Regulation 3). Local authority foster parents must be 'approved' according to criteria set out in the regulations. These include:

- referees – two personal references must be submitted and interviews with them arranged (these may be health professionals)
- health checks – details of the prospective foster parent's health (supported by a medical report) and personality must be provided.

Note that a medical examination is not specified but the guidance suggests that health professionals who know the family should be a source of help, especially in interpreting health information and advising on the extent to which the health of the prospective foster parent – or deteriorating health in the case of an established foster parent – may affect their capacity to act (Vol. 3, para. 3.15).

Reviews of foster parents (Regulation 4). Foster parents have to be reviewed at least once a year to assess that they and their household continue to be suitable. In some cases a review of their health may be necessary.

Agreements (health care needs, Regulation 5). Approved foster parents have to sign two agreements. One covers general matters and requires them to give notice of any serious illness affecting the child or any other serious occurrence. The other is more specific and covers agreed arrangements for the care of each individual child including 'the child's state of health and need for health care and surveillance'.

Health-related advice (Regulation 6). Foster parents must be given 'such advice as appears to be needed'. Where appropriate this may include advice from health professionals especially when a child has special health care needs.

Secure accommodation

Secure accommodation is defined in the Act as 'accommodation provided for the purpose of restricting liberty'. This is generally taken to mean any practice or measure which prevents a child from leaving a room or building of his or her own free will (ie a locked room or a behaviour modification unit in a hospital where the regime is designed to restrict liberty). Ultimately, however, the interpretation of the term is a matter to be determined by a court.

Although such accommodation is an important resource it is nevertheless seen as a 'serious step' and a 'last resort' to be taken only after all other alternatives have been comprehensively considered and rejected (Vol. 4, para. 8.10). Unsurprisingly, the Act imposes strict controls on the use of secure accommodation by local authorities (likewise health and education authorities, NHS trusts, residential care homes, nursing homes and mental nursing homes). These are intended to protect children from unnecessary and inappropriate placements and to ensure that administrative decisions are subject to judicial scrutiny. In addition local authorities have a new duty to take reasonable steps to avoid the need for children within their area to be placed in secure accommodation (Schedule 2, para. 7(c)). Voluntary homes and registered children's homes are not allowed to use secure accommodation.

Criteria for restricting liberty

When can secure accommodation be used? Section 25 states that children must not be placed or kept in secure accommodation unless:

- they have a history of absconding and are likely to abscond from other accommodation, and if they do abscond they are likely to suffer significant harm; or
- if they are kept in any other type of accommodation they are likely to injure themselves or others.

The maximum period of detention without a court's authority is 72 hours (either consecutively or in aggregate) within any period of 28 days. Detention for longer than this requires a court order: a first order may last up to three months, subsequent orders up to six months. Procedural and other related aspects of secure accommodation such as the court's powers, age restrictions, notifications and review mechanisms are also dealt with in regulations. These regulations apply to all children except those detailed under the Mental Health Act 1983, although children being assessed under a child assessment order (Section 43) cannot be placed in secure accommodation.

PRACTICE NOTES

Section 25 now applies to children accommodated by health authorities and NHS trusts. This means:

- that these agencies must comply with Section 25 and the Children (Secure Accommodation) Regulations 1991 and Children (Secure Accommodation) (no. 2) Regulations 1991)
- they can apply to court for a secure accommodation order
- a court order is permissive – it enables the child to be detained but does not prevent his or her release if circumstances change
- it is recommended (Vol. 4, para. 8.16) that applications to the court should be authorized at a senior level within the health authority (ie the consultant or other person with line management responsibility for the ward or establishment in which the child is accommodated).

Case studies

Case study 19

Adelaide is six years old. For nearly a year she has been living with Mr and Mrs Bhutta under a private fostering arrangement while her parents (who are married) are studying abroad. Although Adelaide's parents contacted her regularly at the beginning of the placement, for the past two months they have not been in touch at all. Mr and Mrs Bhutta have tried to trace them without success and are very concerned because Adelaide is due to have surgery shortly.

Ben is three years old. He is also fostered under a private arrangement while his mother works abroad. His father, who never married his mother, disappeared well before his birth. Soon after his placement began his foster mother, Clara, took him to the local health centre while she had a check up. He seemed in good health but while chatting with the practice nurse, Dora, Clara revealed that she knew nothing about Ben's medical history. Dora suggested that Ben be medically examined but Clara says that is not necessary and is too busy to arrange it. She says she expects to hear from Ben's mother in two to three months and will discuss it with her then. Although Dora is not concerned at all about Ben's care she does think he should be examined before his mother returns so that a full medical history can be compiled.

1. Who has parental responsibility for Adelaide and Ben?
2. Who has the right to consent to medical examinations and treatment for Adelaide and Ben?
3. If Clara refuses to agree to Ben's medical examination what action should Dora, the practice nurse take?

Solutions

1. When children are privately fostered parental responsibility is not acquired by the foster parents but is retained by the people who had it before the placement began. This means that because Adelaide's parents were married they both automatically have parental responsibility. On the other hand, as regards Ben, only his mother has parental responsibility since his parents were not married and it is assumed that his father never acquired parental responsibility.
2. The right to consent to medical examination and treatment on behalf of a child is part of parental responsibility. So both Adelaide's parents and Ben's mother have the right to consent. But since Adelaide's parents can not be found it is possible for Mr or Mrs Bhutta, as Adelaide's current carers, to give consent instead (by virtue of Section 3(5) of the Children Act which entitles them 'to do what is necessary in all the circumstances of the case for the purpose of safeguarding or promoting' Adelaide's welfare).
3. Dora should contact the local authority so that they can impose a requirement on Clara (under Schedule 8, para. 6) that Ben be examined either as soon as possible or at regular specified periods.

Case study 20

Colin is 15 years old. He has been in and out of trouble ever since he left primary school and was previously the subject of an education supervision order which lapsed several months ago. For the last five weeks Colin has been accommodated by X Health Authority and because of his very disruptive behaviour he has been kept in a behaviour modification unit (a regime which is intended to restrict his liberty) at a hospital for the last 24 hours.

This short period is not considered long enough however and detention for a further seven days at least is recommended. But Colin's parents Mr and Mrs Dawson object very strongly to this idea and his father insists that he has the right to take Colin home immediately because he has never absconded before and is not likely to try to run away from the hospital. He therefore demands that the hospital staff release Colin straight away.

1. Have X Health Authority the right to detain Colin in secure accommodation? If so, for how long?
2. When can a court make a secure accommodation order? Would hospital staff be involved in these proceedings?
3. Can Colin's father take him home when he wants to?

4. What difference would it make if Colin was subject to a care order?
5. What difference would it make if Colin was on remand or detained in criminal proceedings?

Solutions

1. Statutory safeguards governing the restriction of children's liberty have been extended to children accommodated by health authorities, NHS trusts and in residential care homes, nursing homes and mental nursing homes. Basically, this means that, provided strict criteria (as in Section 25) are met, they cannot be detained in secure accommodation for longer than 72 hours, either consecutively or in aggregate within any period of 28 consecutive days without court authority.

   Colin cannot be kept in secure accommodation unless he has a history of absconding and is likely to abscond from any other type of accommodation and, if he does abscond, be likely to suffer significant harm; or he is likely to injure himself or others if kept in any other type of accommodation. So, providing it appears that Colin is likely to injure himself or others it is immaterial whether or not he has absconded before.

2. Before a court can make a secure accommodation order in respect of Colin it must be satisfied that the criteria in Section 25 apply. In addition, the principles in Section 1 of the Act must be applied and Colin's welfare must be the paramount consideration. No order should be made unless this would be better for Colin than no order at all (the non-intervention principle). Health professionals who have been involved in Colin's care may be asked to advise on the need for an order and its likely effect.

3. As Colin's father has parental responsibility, and Colin is being voluntarily accommodated, he can remove Colin at any time unless there is a residence order in force, in which case he can only be removed with the agreement of the person named in the order. If it is considered necessary to retain him emergency measures such as an emergency protection order would have to be obtained.

4. If Colin was subject to a care order the way his parents exercise parental responsibility would be controlled by the local authority who share parental responsibility whilst the care order is in force. Only, therefore, if the local authority agreed to Colin being removed could he be taken home.

5. If Colin was on remand or detained in criminal proceedings then he could be kept in secure accommodation if he was otherwise likely to abscond or injure himself and others. The fact that he is likely to abscond is sufficient to justify restricting his liberty. There is no need to prove the likelihood of significant harm.

11

Children With Disabilities

This chapter focuses mainly on the Children Act together with an outline of related legislation, notably the Education Act 1981, the Disabled Persons (Services, Consultation and Representation) Act 1986 and the Chronically Sick and Disabled Persons Act 1970.

It is estimated that in Great Britain there are approximatly 360 000 children under 16 with one or more disabilities, representing just over 3% of all children. The Children Act attempts to provide a new legal framework for such children who are, for the first time, specifically included in children's legislation. The reasons for this major reform are twofold. First, to encourage integration of service provision for all children and ensure that those with disabilities are treated as 'children first', with common needs for care, affection and a stimulating environment, and disabled second, with access to a range of generic and specialist provision. Secondly, to ensure that the protections and benefits of child care law apply broadly to all children regardless of which agency is looking after them or providing services.

The Children Act

The intention behind the new framework is that in the context of the Children Act, work with children with disabilities should be based on six fundamental principles. These are:

1. The welfare of the child should be safeguarded and promoted by those providing services.
2. A primary aim should be to promote access for all children to the same range of services.
3. Children with disabilities are children first.
4. Recognition of the importance of parents and families in children's lives.
5. Partnership between parents and local authorities and other agencies.
6. The view of children and parents should be sought and taken into account (Vol. 6, para. 1.6).

To support these principles the Act adopts a number of approaches. Disabled children are included within the general definition of children in need. This means that children who are affected by physical disability, chronic sickness, mental disability, sensory disability, communication impairment, and mental illness must be provided with services under Part III of the Act (*see* Chapter 5). In addition the Act contains various provisions which are specifically 'targeted' at children with disabilities (*see* below). Before looking at these (and other relevant aspects of the Act), the expected overall contribution by child health services will be summarized.

PRACTICE NOTES

The guidance states the role of local social services cannot be fully implemented without close partnership with child health services and shared arrangements for the transfer of information about children and joint planning for their futures (Vol. 6, para. 10.1). In particular the following recommendations are made.

1. Steps should be taken to ensure that medical information is collated and interpreted for the benefit of the child and the family (by forging links between GPs, paediatricians and other specialist medical services).
2. The child health service should ensure that appropriate referrals are made to paramedical services, which in turn can support children's integration into local services.
3. There should be active social services department involvement in, and representation on, child development/district handicap teams and community mental handicap or learning disability teams.
4. Close liaison between social services departments and their child health service counterparts should be established so as to encourage parents to share in recording their children's development and health care needs and to enable them and their children to contribute to decision-making.
5. Social services departments should create links with local child-development centres or teams and any other services which work directly with a wide range of families.

Aspects of the Act which are particularly relevant to children with disabilities are considered below.

Identification and assessment of children 'in need'

Local authorities have important new functions in respect of the identification and assessment of children in need (*see* Part III, Chapter 5). This means they must identify the numbers and needs of children in their area who are disabled through physical, sensory or learning disablement, mental disorders and chronic illness and also consider their overall development needs: physical, social, intellectual, emotional and behavioural. Note that this process is expected to include not just a functional 'MOT-style' assessment but a full 'holistic' assessment which takes into account environmental, social and other related factors.

Moreover, since children with disabilities may need services throughout their lives, the guidance recommends that assessment should be an on-going process, which takes a longer perspective than is usual or necessary and which involves an initial assessment, a continuous reassessment and review.

PRACTICE NOTES

Health professionals are expected to play a key role in identification and assessment procedures, most notably in the following areas:

- liaising with social services departments so as to achieve an understanding of disability which permits early identification and facilitates joint working
- initiating discussions with parents about services and procedures which might be beneficial (if they are the first to identify a child in need)
- developing clear assessment procedures within agreed criteria which take account of the child's and family's needs and preferences, racial and ethnic origins, culture, religion and any special needs, and the power given to local authorities to arrange assessments of disabled children (which can include health and education services)
- ensuring that children with disabilities are treated as children first and thus have access to the same services for health surveillance and promotion as are available to children generally.

Additional services for children with disabilities

Local authorities have a duty to provide services for children with disabilities which are designed to minimize the effects of their disabilities and to give them the opportunity to lead lives that are as normal as possible (Schedule 2, para. 6).

In interpreting this provision local authorities have considerable discretion but the intention is that these extra services should help in the identification, diagnosis, assessment and treatment of children with disabilities and also help them to overcome limitations of mobility and communication. Services which might be relevant in this context include domiciliary services, befriending schemes, family centres and day care provision.

PRACTICE NOTES

Health professionals may be required to help ensure appropriate services are available, especially if they enable children to live at home. For example:

- providing skill and expertise in establishing a home care service such as the Portage home teaching scheme

- facilitating the integration of children with disabilities in the community by ensuring those with special health care needs are not automatically excluded from local children's services
- advising how family centres can best be designed, and offering their services.

Register of children with disabilities

To encourage more coherent planning and monitoring of service provision, the Act requires local authorities to keep a register of children with disabilities. Registration is voluntary on the part of parents and children and is not a pre-condition of service provision. Registers have not generally been very successful previously, having suffered from a fairly negative image and the fact that there is no guarantee of service provision under the Chronically Sick and Disabled Persons Act 1970 (*see* below). They have also in the past been confused with child protection registers.

PRACTICE NOTES

Inter-agency collaboration and co-operation in establishing and maintaining registers is essential if services and assessments are to be co-ordinated and effective. In particular the guidance makes the following recommendations:

- clear criteria for definitions of disability must be agreed
- a joint register should be established between health education and social services
- decisions about registration should not be made when parents and children are suffering emotional stress (for example, when the child's potential disability or special need is first identified)
- counselling provided should be sensitive to individual racial, cultural, linguistic, religious needs or communication difficulties
- confidentiality about individual children and families must be maintained, and appropriate procedures agreed and developed for sharing and transferring information
- in some cases it may be appropriate for a health authority to maintain and operate the register on behalf of a local authority (the responsibility for the register will remain with the local authority however).

Accommodation

To ensure that the special care needs of disabled children are taken into account the Act specifically requires local authorities to make sure that so far as is reasonably practicable, any accommodation provided is 'not unsuitable' for their particular needs (Section 23(8)). This provision should be read alongside other provisions regulating placement, ie that siblings should be accommodated together and children should preferably live with relatives or friends and be placed near their families. Overall, however, the guidance stresses that planning a placement for children with disabilities should follow the same principles as apply to other children. In other words placements should provide permanence, security and an experience of ordinary family life. In addition, contact between children, their parents, relatives and friends and anyone else connected with them is expected to be encouraged (*see* also Chapter 9).

Chapter 11 of Volume 6 gives further guidance on accommodation but the following aspects are especially relevant to health professionals.

Respite care

Short-term care (often called respite care, phased care or family link schemes) has historically developed as an emergency service to meet a family crisis. Now, however, flexible, short-term care which can offer an 'age appropriate local service, compatible with the child's family background, culture and racial origin' is considered preferable.

Foster care

In the last decade there has been a major growth in foster placements for children with a range of special needs. These placements are considered particularly beneficial to children with disabilities since they provide an opportunity for them to grow up in a family setting. Accordingly the guidance urges positive policies on recruitment, training and support programmes which should include opportunities to meet children with disabilities and their parents. It also recommends that the possibility of involving people with disabilities as foster parents or as contributors to training programmes should be actively considered.

Residential care (health establishments)

Although some children with disabilities or with serious health problems may have to spend substantial periods of time receiving care or treatment in an NHS facility, they are not expected to live in hospital settings on a long-term basis. As the guidance stresses 'NHS facilities should reflect a child's need for assessment, treatment or other service which cannot otherwise be provided and should in no way constitute a permanent placement' (Vol. 6, para. 13.7). Nevertheless, where NHS provision is required the aim should be to provide care in small homely, locally-based units.

PRACTICE NOTES

Health professionals may be involved in implementing these recommendations, notably:

- in identifying the particular health needs of individual children and the extent to which they should be met in a health setting; in many instances advice from child health services, with appropriate support, should enable children to continue to be cared for in social services department or voluntary provision
- in increasing the use of foster placements by providing specialist training and advice and information on the nature and the most effective management of a disability.

Complaints procedures

Children with disabilities are most likely to use complaint procedures to challenge assessment and the delivery of (or failure to deliver) certain services.

PRACTICE NOTES

Health professionals may be involved in the following aspects:

- consideration of a complaint – given the multi-professional support needed by many children with disabilities, consideration of a complaint may require consultation with a wide range of relevant expert opinion
- advice and support – professional expertise may be required in framing or pursuing a complaint, especially where a complainant is vulnerable and unsupported or has a complex communication disorder.

Health professionals involved in complaints procedures should be aware of possible conflicts of interest between a child and other persons involved in the dispute, eg the child's parent or other person who may have lodged the complaint on the child's behalf.

Transition to adulthood

The Act imposes new duties to prepare young people for independent adult life. This involves preparation for leaving care by enabling the young to build and maintain relationships with others, developing their self-esteem and teaching them practical and financial skills and knowledge as well as providing after-care services. For some young people with disabilities these duties are especially important since they may have been over-protected and not provided with the same opportunities to develop independence as non-disabled adolescents. In many cases, too, they may need more ongoing care and support than their non-disabled peers.

PRACTICE NOTES

The following specific recommendations may have implications for health professionals (Vol. 6, Chapter 16):

1. *Changes in collaborative working practices.* Planning for post-school provision should take account of a young person's wider personal and social, health, occupational, vocational and educational abilities and needs and may necessitate strengthening and reviewing existing collaborative mechanisms such as district handicap or child development teams, community mental handicap or learning disability teams and joint consultative committees.
2. *Support of primary health team.* In order to ensure that joint planning is followed by joint service arrangements, social services departments are encouraged to have 'precise arrangements for working with district health authorities, family health services authorities and NHS Trusts (where appropriate)'.
3. *Residential provision.* With the cessation of admissions to long-stay hospitals for residential care, social services departments are expected to consider 'as a matter of urgency' how they work in partnership with their health and education counterparts in developing new patterns of residential services which provide good quality care in the local community.

The Chronically Sick and Disabled Persons Act 1970

The Act (CSDPA) was supposed to help disabled people live reasonably independent lives, preferably in their own homes. Unfortunately, however, it has not been very successful, largely because of chronic underfunding and lack of 'legal teeth'. Nevertheless it remains the foundation for local authority services and facilities for disabled people of all ages, including children with disabilities as defined in the Children Act (ie children 'in need' under section 17(10)).

The CSDPA requires local authorities to identify the number of disabled people in its area; to publish information about services available (*see* below) and to ensure that anyone using services is told about other relevant services (*see* also Schedule 2, Part 1 of the Children Act).

In addition, local authorities must make arrangements for the provision of a range of services if they are satisfied that a need exists. These are:

- practical assistance in the home
- provision or assistance in obtaining a radio, television, library or similar recreational facilities

- lectures, games, outings or other recreational facilities outside the home, or assistance in taking advantage of educational facilities
- facilities for, or assistance in, travelling to and from home
- home adaptations (or additional facilities) for greater safety, comfort or convenience
- facilitating holidays
- meals
- provision, or assistance in obtaining a telephone, or equipment to make use of one.

The Disabled Persons (Services, Consultation and Representation) Act 1986

This Act (commonly referred to as the Disabled Persons Act) supplements the provisions of the CSDPA and also applies to both disabled children and adults. Under Section 2 local authorities have to assess the need for services under the CSDPA. Other provisions, notably Sections 5 and 6 are intended to make the process of leaving school for the adult world smoother. Accordingly, they require authorities to identify disabled school-leavers and assess their need for services. The remaining sections deal with, for example, information about services and the need to take account of the abilities of carers to continue to provide regular care when deciding on the need for services.

The Act also aims to strengthen the notion of entitlement to services specified under the CSDPA and to provide disabled people with a stronger voice. However, some of its provisions will not now be implemented as they have been superseded by the community care provisions and the Children Act.

Note also, that at 18, young people who have a continuing need for community care services, or who may require them for the first time, are covered by the provisions of the NHS and Community Care Act 1990, which include an assessment of their need for services.

The Education Act 1981

Before 1981 children with disabilities were categorized for educational purposes by a process which was both stigmatizing and discriminatory. As a result they were segregated (and marginalized) in special schools. The Education Act 1981 sought to reverse this process by de-stigmatizing special needs and integrating children with learning difficulties into mainstream education. Accordingly it established legally defined and prescribed procedures in which special needs could be assessed and provided for, preferably in ordinary schools. As a result there are now 20 000 fewer children being educated in special schools than there were ten years ago.

The Act provides that a child has a special education need (SEN) if he or she has a learning difficulty which requires special educational provision. Unfortunately the phrase 'learning difficulty' is defined very imprecisely and relativistically, giving education authorities considerable scope for interpretation. Inevitably, therefore, there are wide variations in the way the term is interpreted in practice, likewise in the extent of, and provision for, special education needs.

In summary, the strategy of integration adopted by the Act consists of ensuring that children with SEN are identified and appropriately assessed and, if necessary, reassessed so that the nature of their needs can be understood and a decision can be made about additional, or different, educational provision. If it is decided that a special need does exist the education authority must issue a 'statement' of the relevant needs and arrange for the special educational provision, unless suitable arrangements are made by the children's parents. 'Statements', which must be reviewed annually, are formal documents whose form and contents are prescribed by regulations. However, the proportion of 'statemented' children differs widely between authorities.

A key feature of the Act is the way it attempts to involve parents by, for example, giving them rights to initiate assessments, to comment and be consulted and to appeal. But unfortunately, given the complexity of the assessment and statementing processes and the extensive case law the Act has generated, it seems that only the 'most articulate of parents' have benefited from these provisions.

PRACTICE NOTES

The Children Act has strengthened the legal framework regarding co-operation between authorities in order to foster a co-ordinated support network for children with SENs. Health professionals are, however, most likely to be involved in the following:

Identification and notification. Early identification of a SEN is considered crucial for young children with disabilities. Hence:

1. Section 10 of the Education Act 1981 requires district health authorities to notify parents and education authorities of any children under five who might have a SEN. In addition, health authorities must provide parents of such children with information about any voluntary organization which might be useful, for example, to provide counselling.

2. Education circular 22/89 highlights four particular cases when health authorities should consider initiating an assessment of a child's potential SENs. These are:

- if the child has a medical condition likely to affect future learning
- if the child has been admitted in connection with a social condition which is likely to affect future learning ability (such as social deprivation, whether negligence, neglect or child abuse)
- if a child is receiving treatment likely to affect future learning ability
- if the child has been admitted to a children's or adolescent psychiatric ward.

Assessment. Various aspects of the 'multifactorial' assessment process (which is governed by detailed regulations) may involve health professionals. In particular:

1. Education authorities must obtain written 'medical and psychological' advice and any other advice they consider desirable in making an assessment. In this context medical advice is to be taken in its widest sense to include co-ordinated concise and relevant information from doctors and other non-medical specialists. They must also take into account any information about a child's health provided by the health authority.

2. Assessments under the Education Act 1981, the Children Act, the Disabled Persons Act 1986 and the Chronically Sick and Disabled Persons Act 1970 can, and should whenever possible, be combined so as to ensure a collaborative, cost-effective and co-ordinated approach.

3. Education authorities can arrange for a child to be medically or otherwise examined for the purposes of assessment.

Statements. Health professionals may be involved in the preparation of the statement of special educational needs. They may also be asked to advise on whether a child could benefit from the new power (introduced by the Children Act) which allows statemented children to go to establishments outside England and Wales, such as the Peto Institute in Hungary.

Case studies

Case study 21

Dawn is just over four years old. She is blind and also has hearing problems. She has only recently moved into the area with her parents and her eight-year-old brother Ethan (the family have just moved to England). Dawn has a serious chest infection and her mother, Elizabeth, takes her to the local health centre. While there she tells the GP and health visitor that she is finding it very difficult to cope with Dawn. Without lots of support she is worried that she will not be able to look after her at home for much longer, especially as she is now also very concerned about Ethan's poor progress at school. In fact Elizabeth is due to see his teacher in a couple of days to discuss his problems, especially his difficulties.

1. Are Dawn or Ethan entitled to local authority support services?
2. What assessments are likely to be made of the children?
3. Must Elizabeth co-operate in the assessment procedures before services can be provided?
4. What should be done if the GP thinks that Dawn needs a detailed assessment but Elizabeth refuses to arrange an appointment?

Solutions

1. Dawn could be defined as a child 'in need' as she is blind and clearly comes within the definition of 'disabled' in Section 17(10) of the Children Act. Whether Ethan could be defined as also 'in need' would depend on whether he was considered 'unlikely to achieve or maintain, or have the opportunity of achieving or maintaining, a reasonable standard of health or development without the provision of services; or whether his health or development was likely to be significantly, or further impaired, without the provision of services'.

   As a 'disabled' child Dawn could benefit from a wide range of services some of which are specificallly designed to minimize the effects of her disability and enable her to lead as normal a life as possible. For example, befriending schemes or domiciliary services might be especially useful. Dawn's name could also be entered on the register of children with disabilities, although Elizabeth's refusal to agree to this would not affect Dawn's entitlement to services.

   If Ethan was considered 'in need' he, too, might benefit from services, such as after-school activities (he may even be provided with these if not 'in need').
2. Local authorities must identify children in need in order to assess what services they should provide. However the Children Act enables assessments under the Education Act 1981 (to establish 'special educational need') to be combined with other assessments, such as those under the Children Act itself and the Chronically Sick and Disabled Persons Act 1970, assessments which might be relevant both for Dawn and Ethan.
3. Elizabeth is not obliged either to co-operate in the assessment procedures or to accept services. However, her refusal may be significant if at some later date there is anxiety about the children's welfare.
4. If Elizabeth cannot be persuaded to let Dawn be assessed, for example, she makes appointments but repeatedly fails to keep them, a child assessment order could be applied for by the local authority unless there were urgent concerns about Dawn's welfare in which case an emergency protection order would be more appropriate.

12

Adoption

Adoption is a process which legally transfers a child from one family group to another. Aptly described as a 'legal transplant' it completely severs the legal relationship between a child and his or her natural parents and transfers all parental responsibility to the adoptive parent, who for all legal purposes then replace the child's natural parents. Adoption is the only way parental responsibility can be entirely transferred during the parents' lifetime.

Although adoption has declined steadily in the last two decades, from a peak of nearly 25 000 in 1968 to just over 7000 in 1989, it is increasingly seen as an acceptable long-term option for many children in care, especially those who are said to be 'hard' to place such as older children or those with special needs. Unsurprisingly, adoption is also seen as an appropriate way of achieving permanency and security for children whose links with their 'birth family' have broken down. As such adoption is now a significant element of child care practice.

Adoption law was excluded from the extensive review process which preceded the Children Act because it has been the subject of its own separate review (*see* below). Some amendments to existing laws have been made by the Act however, although these are generally not substantive. The law of adoption is contained in the Adoption Act 1976, regulations and court rules. It is detailed and complex and involves a two stage procedure. The first is the internal agency procedure and the second is the court application. In summary, the adoption process is as follows:

The role of adoption services and agencies

Investigations

The Adoption Act 1976 requires all local authorities to set up and maintain a comprehensive adoption service. This can be provided either directly by the local authority – acting through their social services departments – or by approved adoption societies (both are referred to as adoption agencies). The work and duties of adoption agencies are prescribed in the Adoption Agency Regulations 1983. Broadly these require agencies to carry out extensive investigations, obtain reports and provide counselling. In addition they must ascertain the child's wishes and feelings and consider the parents' wishes about religious upbringing. Further consultation duties are imposed by the Children Act (*see* Sections 22 and 61 and Chapter 9). Detailed information about the child and his or her parents, including full health histories, must also be gathered and arrangements made for medical examinations and so on. They must also fully investigate the prospective adopters.

PRACTICE NOTES

Health professionals may be involved in various examinations and reports which the British Agencies for Adoption and Fostering recommend be completed. Although not all of these are statutorily required they are in universal use throughout child care agencies. They are as follows:

Reports on children. They include:

- a neonatal report (to provide the placing agency with information about a baby who is to be discharged from hospital to prospective adopters)
- summary retrospective report from paediatric and/or maternity record (to meet the placement needs of older children, for when full neonatal records may no longer be readily available)
- preliminary report on a child to be looked after (to provide carers with adequate medical information)
- medical history card (to provide an ongoing record of the child's medical history)
- medical reports and development assessment of a child under five and aged five to ten (to encourage the collation of all relevant medical information on the child and background information which may be relevant when the child is older)
- profile of behavioural and emotional well-being of a child aged one to five and five to ten (to make use of the current carer's knowledge, day-to-day observation and understanding of the child)
- medical report and functional assessment of a young person aged 11 and over
- annual medical report on a child or young person in foster care
- health passport (to encourage young people to take an interest in and eventually take responsibility for their own health care).

Reports on adults. These include:

- medical report on birth parents (to obtain background health information which will assist in deciding on the best placement for the child)
- obstetric report on the mother (to provide information about the health of the mother before, during, and after delivery)
- medical report on the prospective adoptive parent (to obtain an accurate, up-to-date report, based on medical examination and medical facts from records, on the applicant's individual and family health history and current physical and mental health)
- update of medical report on prospective adoptive parent.

Adoption panel

The panel which includes social workers, a medical adviser, and at least two independent members must consider all the information gathered by the adoption agency and make recommendations as to whether prospective adopters are suitable, whether they would be suitable for the particular child, and whether adoption is in the child's best interests. Essentially, therefore, the panel is involved in a 'matching process', the broad aim of which is to ensure that the adopted child 'fits in' with his or her new family.

Placement

If the adoption panel decides that a proposed adoption should go ahead and the agency accepts its recommendations – which it is not bound to do – the placement can proceed. Procedure at this point is, however, governed by complex provisions which, amongst other things, include notification requirements as well as various supervisory duties (ie visiting).

It is perhaps worth noting that although the vast majority of placements are arranged through adoption agencies it is still possible for private individuals to arrange placements. But these are now very rare, mainly because they are prohibited except in some circumstances. When they are arranged, however, local authorities must be notified and are then obliged to carry out various investigative and reporting duties.

Eligibility

Who can be adopted?

To be adopted a child must be unmarried and under 18 (an adopted child can be re-adopted).

Who can adopt?

The Adoption Act 1976 permits both joint and sole applications. In practice most adoptions are by married couples – a significant number being 'step-parent adoptions' – where a parent, usually the mother, and a new spouse, who is not the child's parent, jointly apply to adopt the child. Joint applications are not allowed unless the applicants are married. This means, therefore, that cohabiting couples cannot adopt.

Sole applicants are likely to be relatives or an unmarried parent of the child. In the past it was not uncommon for unmarried mothers to adopt their own children as a way of hiding their illegitimacy.

The law also lays down age restrictions. Applicants must be at least 21, or 18 if the applicant is a natural parent, but there is no upper age limit. However, one may be imposed in practice.

Parental consent

In principle no adoption order can be made unless the child's natural parents (or guardians) consent. If the child's parents are not married, the father's consent is only required if he has acquired parental responsibility and a mother's consent is not effective until six weeks after her child's birth. All consents must be given freely and unconditionally with a full understanding of what is involved. If parents refuse consent courts can dispense with their agreement, in which case the court will appoint a guardian ad litem to protect the child's interests.

The Adoption Act (Section 16) sets out six grounds for dispensing with consent. These are that the parent or guardian:

- cannot be found or is incapable of giving agreement
- is withholding agreement unreasonably
- has persistently failed without reasonable cause to discharge parental responsibility for the child
- has abandoned or neglected the child
- has persistently ill-treated the child
- has seriously ill-treated the child (and rehabilitation in the parents' household is unlikely).

Freeing for adoption

A major flaw in adoption law used to be the possibility that a parent could only consent to a specific adoption which could be withdrawn at any time before the adoption order was made. The chance that parents might change their minds was a major cause of anxiety to prospective adopters. This led to a change in the law in 1984 and since then it has been possible for an adoption agency to get a court order 'freeing' a child for adoption. This procedure effectively 'stamps' the child as free for adoption and transfers parental responsibility to the adoption agency. Importantly it also means that the parents do not have to consent to a specific adoption application. Instead their general consent is given and the child is in effect 'placed on a shelf to await suitable adopters', although it could be months or even years before the child is actually adopted.

Legal status of children placed for adoption (or pre-adoption foster placements)

Before the Children Act some children awaiting adoption (usually babies) were subject only to the adoption agencies' regulations and their legal status was uncertain. Now all children placed by agencies are subject to the relevant provisions of the Children Act (likewise the Adoption Regulations). This means that for local authorities such children will be included within the definition of 'looked after' (whether they are in care as a result of a care order, voluntarily accommodated or have been freed for adoption; *see* Secton 22 and Chapter 9 for the range of duties owed to them).

All children placed for adoption are subject to the Arrangement and Review Regulations 1991. This means that they must be medically examined and assessed at the time of placement, unless this was done within the previous three months and follow-up examinations are carried out (*see* Chapter 9).

Court procedure

A court order is always required for adoption. This gives the court a chance to ensure that the adoption is in the child's best interests and that parental consent has been obtained or dispensed with. But no order can be made until the child has lived with the prospective adopters for specified periods. The periods vary depending on who is proposing to adopt and who made the original placement. These periods are supposed to give the child time to settle down and the proposed adopters time to adjust to their new parental role. They also give time for the placement to be assessed. The Adoption Act prohibits an order being made unless the court is satisfied that there have been sufficient opportunities to see the child with the prospective adopters in the 'home environment'.

In reaching any decision the court is bound to have regard to all the circumstances and to give first consideration to the need to safeguard and promote the welfare of the child throughout his or her childhood. It must also take into account the child's wishes and feelings and give due consideration to them, according to his or her age and understanding. To help a court reach a decision various detailed reports must be considered.

If the court is satisifed that adoption is the most appropriate option it will make the order. From then on the child is treated as if it were the legitimate child of the adoptive parents except for certain purposes (these relate to citizenship, marriage and incest laws). If adoption is considered inappropriate, various alternatives are possible. These include an interim order (this gives the adoptive parents parental responsibility for a probationary period of two years), residence or other Section 8 orders or no order at all.

Adoption allowances

Adoption allowances were first introduced in 1982 on an individual experimental basis. Since it seemed that they significantly increased the adoption of hard-to-place children they were retained and are now governed by the Adoption Allowance Regulations 1991. The main 'beneficiaries' of the allowance scheme are children with special needs but to qualify they must come within specified criteria, which in itself does not guarantee payment.

PRACTICE NOTES

Health professionals may be asked to help evaluate children and assess whether they fit the relevant criteria set out in Regulation 2 – whether they are mentally or physically disabled, or suffering from the effects of emotional or behavioural difficulties, and need special care which requires greater expenditure of resources than would be required if they were not so disabled or suffering from the effects of emotional or behavioural difficulties.

In particular the role of health professionals is expected to be of 'special value' in evaluating the degree of a child's condition and in providing relevant advice to adoption agencies and adoptive parents (Vol. 9, para. 2.28).

Tracing origins (The Adoption Contact Register)

In the past it was thought best that adopted children's break from their birth families should be total. Unsurprisingly, therefore, the adoption process was closed and secretive and designed to deliberately 'fix a gulf between a child's past and future'. But studies in the 1960s and 70s revealed the importance of children knowing their own identities and keeping or establishing contact with their birth families. The law was therefore changed in 1975 and since then adopted adults over 18 have been entitled to see their original birth records. This has enabled some adopted people to trace and make contact with their birth parents and other relatives, although it did not guarantee that such contact would be welcome.

Accordingly, the Children Act establishes a new Adoption Contact Register, the purpose of which is to provide a safe and confidential way to put adopted people in touch with their birth parents and other relatives where it is what they both want. This register has the potential to provide much more information than can be obtained from a birth certificate although it cannot help an adopted person discover the whereabouts of his or her birth parent or other relative unless that person has chosen to be entered on the register (*see* Vol. 9, Chapter 3).

Reform of adoption law

One of the reasons why adoption law has not been more substantially reformed by the Children Act is that the existing system is currently being reviewed. The impetus for change is partly due to the changing patterns of adoption. For example, an increasing proportion of adoptions are made in respect of older children, for whom the severing of links with their birth families may be neither desirable nor possible. The number of children adopted from care has also risen in recent years, as have inter-country adoptions.

But perhaps the most important issue to emerge in the review process is the concept of openness. It has been suggested, for example, that adoption law and practice should attempt to promote greater consultation among all interested parties and, where appropriate, increased exchange of information. Continued post-adoption contact between adopted children and their birth families is also an issue of concern, likewise the related issue of giving birth parents a right to information about their child after adoption. Another major area of proposed change – which is potentially very important given the increasing willingness of agencies to consider adoption in spite of parental opposition – centres around the criteria for dispensing with parental agreement.

Reform of adoption is likely to occur reasonably quickly but since many of the proposals could have far-reaching implications, further detailed study is necessary. In the meantime reforms introduced by the Children Act will considerably increase the court's powers in adoption proceedings, notably because Section 8 orders (residence, contact, prohibited steps and specific issue orders) can be made in adoption proceedings.

13

Challenging Local Authorities

Disputes about children can arise in a number of different contexts in the public law system. They may centre on the Part III provision or relate to the treatment of a child being looked after by a local authority. Alternatively compulsory measures may be the cause of complaint. To deal with these kinds of disputes various options are available (apart from appeals procedures) which enable parents and others to challenge the way a local authority has acted or failed to act. A summary of these follows.

Complaints procedure

Local authorities, likewise voluntary organizations and registered children's homes, have a duty to establish a procedure for considering representations and complaints (Section 26). Complaints can be made about any aspect of their Part III functions. This includes the provision of services and the way children are looked after (whether on a voluntary basis or as a result of compulsory intervention). The potential range of complaints is thus very broad, it can involve relatively minor grievances or major ones such as the kind of accommodation provided, day care services, quality of social work support, proposed medical treatment, change of placement and so on. The decision-making process itself could also be the basis of a complaint that the child or his or her parents were not consulted or given adequate information.

A wide range of people can invoke the complaints procedure, including the child, his or her parents, those with parental responsibility, foster parents and anyone whom the local authority considers has sufficient interest in the child's welfare.

PRACTICE NOTES

Health professionals may well be involved in the consideration of a complaint, especially if it concerns family support or child protection work to which they have contributed.

A health professional may be the most appropriate person to initiate a complaint, for example to register opposition to proposed medical or psychiatric examination or treatment.

Judicial review

Local authority decisions can also be challenged by judicial review. This procedure can only be invoked if it can be shown that an authority has misdirected itself in law, acted unlawfully or unreasonably (irrationally or perversely) or failed to consider relevant matters. Failure to observe proper procedures or breaching rules of natural justice, ie not giving a person a chance to state their case, may also justify an application.

Other avenues of complaint

Complaints about maladministration within local government may also be made to the Commissioner for Local Administration (Ombudsman). In addition the Secretary of State also has various powers and can set up inquiries or make default orders. As a last resort a complaint can be made to the European Court of Human Rights.

The role of wardship

Under previous law local authorities used wardship (a non-statutory procedure) whenever they considered their statutory powers inadequate or inappropriate. Wardship was a means of dodging or bypassing existing statutory grounds for compulsory intervention. It could not, however, be effectively used against local authorities as a means of reviewing, challenging or questioning their decisions. This 'imbalance' was considered untenable, unfair and illogical and not surprisingly the Children Act restricts the use of wardship (likewise the court's inherent jurisdiction) by or in favour of local authorities. The court's inherent jurisdiction is very similar to wardship in that it allows the court to resolve disputes about children (but does not involve the court in any continuing supervision). In summary, the broad effect of the restrictions is to make wardship, the inherent jurisdiction and local authority care incompatible. In particular Section 100 states:

1. Neither wardship nor the inherent jurisdiction can be used to place a child in the care of or under the supervision of a local authority. Neither can they be used so as to require the child to be accommodated by or on behalf of a local authority. This means that if a local authority wants to supervise, take over or retain the care of a child it must use the statutory powers conferred by the Act (Parts IV and V).

2. Wardship (likewise the inherent jurisdiction) cannot be used so as to give a local authority the power to make parental decisions in respect of a child. This means that a court cannot confer on a local authority any degree of parental responsibility it does not already have.

3. A child subject to a care order cannot be made a ward of court.

4. A local authority can, as a last resort, use the court's inherent jurisdiction to resolve an issue concerning the future of a child in its care. But it must get the court's leave (the leave criteria are very stringent) which is only likely to be granted when highly contentious decisions need to be made and/or those which fall outside the normal scope of decision-making.

PRACTICE NOTES

Medical treatment. A local authority may seek the court's approval for certain controversial health-related decisions about a child in care, for example abortion, sterilization or the continuation of life-support treatment. If so, professional health expertise may be sought.

Appendix A

Children Act Guidance Volumes

1. Court Orders

2. Family Support, Day Care and Educational Provision for Young Children

3. Family Placements

4. Residential Care

5. Independent Schools

6. Children with Disabilities

7. Guardians ad Litem and other Court Related Issues

8. Private Fostering and Miscellaneous

9. Adoption Issues

Appendix B

The Abortion Act 1967

Abortions are illegal unless they are carried out in accordance with the provisions of the Abortion Act 1967. This states that a pregnancy can be terminated by a doctor if two doctors have decided in good faith, that the grounds specified in the Act exist. These grounds are:

1. That the pregnancy has not exceeded its 24th week and the continuation of the pregnancy would involve risk of injury to the woman's health (physical or mental), or that of any of her existing children in her family, greater than if the pregnancy were terminated
2. That the termination is necessary to prevent grave permanent injury to the woman's health (physical or mental), or
3. That the continuation of the pregnancy would involve risk to the life of the pregnant woman, greater than if the pregnancy were terminated, or
4. That there is a substantial risk that the child would be seriously handicapped owing to physical or mental abnormalities.

In assessing the risks involved in grounds 1 and 2 account can be taken of the woman's actual or reasonably foreseeable environment.

In emergencies – where termination is immediately necessary to save the life or to prevent grave permanent injury to the woman's health (physical or mental) – the requirement to satisfy two doctors is relaxed and one doctor can act alone.

Other provisions of the Act worth noting are the 'conscience clause' which gives conscientious objectors the legal right to refuse to take part in abortions (except when their participation is required to save the life or to prevent grave permanent injury to the physical or mental health of a pregnant woman).

Note also, that it is now clear that selective reduction of pregnancy (ie termination of one or more, but not all fetuses in a multiple pregnancy) may be performed provided the criteria in the Abortion Act are met (but not otherwise).

Appendix C

Growing up: age requirements

Rights given to young people increase with age. The following is a brief summary of some of the age restrictions imposed by law. Others relating to medical treatment are dealt with in detail in Chapter 3.

At any age

Children can:

- be made wards of court
- initiate proceedings under the Children Act 1989 (if they have sufficient understanding)
- choose their religion (unless harmful)
- apply to see most personal files
- sue in court (through a 'next friend')
- make and be bound by certain contracts for such things as food and employment
- open a bank account
- inherit property
- formally complain about race or sexual discrimination
- smoke (unless stopped by a uniformed policeman or park-keeper who have a duty to seize tobacco or cigarette papers (but not pipes or tobacco pouches) from any child apparently under 16 smoking in any street or public place).

At five

Children can:

- drink alcohol in private (under that age alcohol consumption is allowed only on doctor's orders or in an emergency)
- see a U or PG film unaccompanied (at the cinema manager's discretion)

and must

- receive full-time education at school or elsewhere.

At seven

Children can open and draw money from a National and Trustee Savings Bank Account.

At ten

Children can:

- be convicted of a crime (if it can be proved they knew what they were doing was wrong)
- be searched, finger-printed, photographed (and have samples taken) by the police
- be detained 'during Her Majesty's pleasure' for a specified period if guilty of homicide.

At 12

Children can:

- buy a pet
- be trained to take part in dangerous performances.

At 13

Children can:

- work part-time (but only in certain jobs and subject to various conditions)
- in certain circumstances, be employed by their parents in light agricultural or horticultural work.

At 14

Children can:

- have an air weapon (ie air rifle, gun or pistol), and shot gun
- be convicted of rape or other offences involving sexual intercourse
- work part-time as a street trader (subject to certain conditions)
- drive and ride in an agricultural tractor or machine
- go into a pub but not buy or drink alcohol
- be convicted of a criminal offence as if an adult (although sentence and trial are different).

At 15

Children can:

- open a Giro account (with a guarantor)
- see a category 15 film
- if boys, be sent to prison (in certain circumstances).

At 16

Young people can:

- leave school and work full-time (but not, for example in a bar, other licensed premises or betting shop)
- leave home (with parental consent)
- probably leave home without parental consent (but if considered at risk action may be taken, for example, care proceedings)
- marry with parental consent (or the court's permission)
- join a trade union
- if a girl, legally consent to sexual intercourse (a boy can consent at any age)
- apply for a passport (with a parent's consent) and be deleted from a parent's passport
- buy cigarettes, tobacco, cigarette papers, explosives (including fireworks) and liqueur chocolates
- drink beer, porter, cider or perry with a meal in the dining area of a pub or hotel
- buy premium bonds
- enter and live in a brothel (this is also allowed up to the age of four but not between four and 16)
- sell scrap metal
- become a street trader
- drive an invalid carriage, moped and certain tractors
- if a boy, join the armed forces (with parental consent)
- get a national insurance number
- be used for begging
- fly solo in a glider
- apply for legal aid, advice and assistance
- claim income support (but only in certain limited circumstances).

At 17

Young people can:

- drive a motorcycle, car or small goods vehicle
- buy or hire a crossbow, any firearm or ammunition
- fly a plane
- apply for a helicopter pilot's licence
- be tried for a criminal offence as an adult.

At 17½

Young people can:

- if a girl, join the armed forces (with parental consent).

At 18

Children reach the age of majority and can do most things, such as:

- vote
- marry (without parental consent)
- serve on a jury
- make a will
- join the armed forces (without parental consent)
- apply for a passport (without parental consent)
- buy and drink alcohol in a bar
- work in a bar
- be tattooed
- own land
- bet and go into a sex shop
- enter into binding contracts
- change their names
- not be made a ward of court
- see a category 18 film
- pawn goods at a pawn shop.

At 21

Young people can:

- stand in a general or local election
- apply for a liquor licence
- if a man, consent to homosexual acts in private (provided both parties are over 21)
- drive a lorry or bus.

Appendix D

Protective legislation

In addition to provisions in the Children Act the law contains numerous other provisions – largely criminal offences against or involving children – designed to protect children from harm. The following is a summary of some of these provisions:

It is an offence to:

- wilfully assult, ill-treat, neglect, abandon or expose children in a manner likely to cause them unnecessary suffering or injury to health
- allow children between the ages of four and 16 into a brothel (the offence is committed by those caring for the children)
- allow someone under 16 to be used for begging
- give alcohol to children under five (except on doctor's orders or in an emergency)
- sell tobacco or cigarette papers to children apparently under 16
- expose children under 12 to the risk of burning (the offence is committed if the child is so exposed and is killed or seriously injured)
- tattoo children under 18
- allow children under 14 to ride a horse on a road without protective headgear
- knowingly sell alcohol (or allow it to be sold) in licensed premises to children under 18 or allow them to drink alcohol in a bar
- sell explosive substances to children apparently under 16, crossbows to children under 17 and firearms to children under 14
- perform any form of circumcision on a female of whatever age, unless medically necessary
- effect any betting transaction with or through children under 18 or to employ such children in a betting office.
- be drunk and in charge of children under seven in any public or licensed premises.

Other criminal offences seek to protect children from harmful publications, pornography, drugs and noxious substances. Further protection is provided by a range of specific sexual offences involving children. These include incest, unlawful intercourse with girls under 16, abduction and indecent assault.

Appendix E

Further reading

Adcock M, White R and Hollows A (1991) *Significant harm*. Significant Publications, London.

Allen N (1992) *Making sense of the Children Act 1989*, 2nd ed. Longman London.

Bainham A (1990) *Children – the new law, the Children Act 1989*. Family Law.

Bridge J, Bridge S and Luke S (1990) *Blackstone's guide to the Children Act*. Blackstone Press Limited, London.

Department of Health (1990) *An introduction to the Children Act 1989*. HMSO, London.

Department of Health (1990) *Principles and practice in regulations and guidance*. HMSO, London.

Department of Health (1990) *Diagnosis of sexual abuse: Guidance for doctors*. HMSO, London.

Department of Health (1991) *Protecting children: A handbook for social workers*. HMSO, London.

Department of Health (1991) *Welfare of children and young people in hospital*. HMSO, London.

Department of Health (1991) *Working together under the Children Act: A guide to arrangements for inter-agency co-operation for the protection of children from abuse*. HMSO, London.

Department of Health (1991) *Guidance and Regulations*, (9 vols). HMSO, London.

Department of Health (1991) *Child abuse: A study of inquiry reports, 1980–89*. HMSO, London.

Department of Health (1991) *Patterns and outcomes in child placement*. HMSO, London.

Department of Health (1992) *Child protection: Guidance for senior nurses, health visitors and midwives*. HMSO, London.

Department of Health (1992) *The Children Act 1989: NHS study pack*. HMSO, London.

Department of Health (1993) *Evaluating the child protection service*. HMSO, London.

Eekelaar J and Dingwall R (1990) *The reform of child care law: A practical guide to the Children Act 1989*. Routledge, London.

Family Rights Group (1991) *Working in partnership with families: Trainers' pack*. HMSO, London.

Family Rights Group (1991) *Working in partnership with families: Participants' pack*. HMSO, London.

Feldman L (1992) *Child protection law*. Longman, London.

Freeman MDA (1992) *Children, their families and the law*. Macmillan, London.

Hallett C and Birchall E (1992) *Coordination and child protection: A review of the literature*. HMSO, London.

Her Majesty's Stationery Office (1993) *Children Act report*. HMSO, London.

Her Majesty's Stationery Office (1993) *Children first: A study of hospital services*. HMSO, London.

Lyon CM (1993) *The law relating to children*. Butterworths, London.

Mallinson I (1992) *The Children Act: A social care guide*. Whiting & Birch Ltd, London.

Masson J and Morris M (1992) *The Children Act manual*. Sweet and Maxwell, London.

Mitchells B and Prince A (1992) *The Children Act and medical practice*. Family Law, London.

Parker R, Ward H, Jackson S and Aldgate J (1991) *Looking after children: assessing outcomes in child care*. HMSO, London.

Robbins D (1990) *Child care: Putting it in writing: A review of English local authorities' child care policy statement*. HMSO, London.

Utting W (1991) *Children in the public care*. HMSO, London.

White R, Carr P and Lowe N (1990) *A guide to the Children Act 1989*. Butterworths, London.

Williams R (ed) (1992) *A concise guide to the Children Act 1989*. Gaskell, London.

Williams R and Hendricks JH (1992) The Children Act 1989. In: Pickersgill D (ed) *The law and general practice*. Radcliffe Medical Press, Oxford.

Index